recharge

A Year of Self-Care to Focus on *You*

JULIE MONTAGU

piatkus

PIATKUS

First published in Great Britain in 2018 by Piatkus

1 3 5 7 9 10 8 6 4 2

A CIP catalogue record for this book
is available from the British Library.

The names of individuals featured in this book
have been changed to protect their privacy

ISBN 978-0-349-41814-8

Illustrations by Harmsworth Fine Stationery
Typeset in Baskerville by M Rules
Printed and bound in Great Britain by
Clays Ltd, St Ives plc

Papers used by Piatkus are from well-managed forests
and other responsible sources.

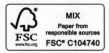

Piatkus
An imprint of
Little, Brown Book Group
Carmelite House
50 Victoria Embankment
London EC4Y 0DZ

An Hachette UK Company
www.hachette.co.uk

www.improvementzone.co.uk

For my husband, Luke

Contents

Acknowledgments

A massive thank-you to the Julie Montagu team – you guys are awesome in every way: Alix Coe, you've been with me now for five years now (can't quite believe it) and always get everything back to me within seconds, even when most of it is on a last-minute deadline; Erica Gellerman, this book would not have happened without your vision for Truly Julie and to offer 'small moments of self-care' to the world; Monique Wassenar, for organising everything and everyone in my life; Stephen Banks, for your patience during the constant photo-taking at Mapperton Estate (all in the name of Instagram) and filming my YouTube videos, but also helping me eat the YouTube recipes; Andrea Raffety, for your support and hard work in making the Julie Montagu School of Yoga dream come true; and Hannah Bryce, the best PR a girl could ask for.

And, of course, last but not least, my four kids – Emma, Jack, William and Nestor: everything I do, I do for you four because you are my everything.

Introduction

Getting to Know *You*

I struggle to find the time to put myself first.

I sacrifice my own self-care because of my –
or my family's – busy lifestyle.

Sound familiar? Well, your struggle stops here, because I know that small moments of self-care lead to big changes. And I know that they can help you. Why?

Well, I have been where you are: busy, tired and letting self-care slip away. Between being a wife, a mother (to four kids) and working, looking after myself wasn't a priority. I was exhausted and I knew I couldn't keep it up for ever. But once I started taking care of myself, everything changed. When I started to prioritise self-care, my energy levels skyrocketed, and I felt strong, healthy and capable.

So what exactly do I mean by self-care? Essentially, it's doing those things that help us to feel good about ourselves. That's unique to each of us, of course, and can range from seemingly small things, such as repeating a positive affirmation to something like participating in a yoga session or meditative practice. It may also take the form of an ongoing exercise regime, caring for your body and mind through healthy eating, spending some time alone with your thoughts and also making the time for meaningful interactions with friends and family.

When you master the art of making self-care a priority, you will not only enhance your physical health but your mental health, too. This is something that is becoming more widely acknowledged by the National Health Service (NHS) in the UK, with self-care programmes being introduced around the country.

With all the demands of a busy, modern-day life, our self-care is often the first thing to go, and the potential negative health implications of this, such as depression, diabetes and obesity, can soon become serious and tricky to reverse. I know that you don't have time to spare to become an expert on everything – that's why I am sharing my experiences and advice with you in easy-to-understand, manageable chunks. My goal is to guide, support and inspire you as you strive to be the happiest, healthiest version of yourself. My health, fitness and well-being advice is specifically designed to be worked into your busy schedule, and will support you on your journey to health and happiness. With an abundance of guidance, tips and easy-to-follow advice, you will find it simple to keep self-care at the forefront of your mind *and* at the top of your to-do list.

The combined pressures of maintaining a balance between our careers and our home and social life can leave many of us feeling as though we aren't doing enough. And this feeling is only exacerbated by social media and the constant barrage of photos, videos and other posts showing how great everyone else has it.

Check your own social feeds now and you will no doubt see a stream of smiling friends with flawless faces, or perhaps photos of their perfectly behaved children, or maybe their beautiful holiday photos in which everyone is having an amazing time. If you look at your own feed, you will probably see similar pictures, but you will know how rare those perfect moments are in among the more usual chaos. And of course, the same is true for everyone else.

Most of us are just so frickin' tired. We're juggling a million and one things, crossing tasks off to-do lists, while adding more at the same time. We are taking care of everything and everyone else, while desperately trying to find the energy to feel good about ourselves until, eventually, we burn out.

Put simply – we need to recharge.

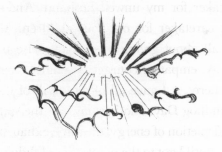

My Self-care Journey

It's taken me many years, and a lot of pain, tears and struggle with self-esteem, self-worth and self-love issues to focus on my self-care. But I can wholeheartedly tell you that it has been worth it.

I didn't wake up one morning and think that I needed to learn more about self-care. I didn't want a degree in it. I simply realised that I needed to start taking care of me, or else I was going to fall into a downward spiral. And if that happened, who would take care of my family? That's where the self-care journey began. My destination? *Me*. Caring for *me*.

January 2009. This was the start of my descent into exhaustion, unhappiness, self-loathing and all that went with it. I was a mother to four small children aged nine, seven, four and two. Oh, and happily married too. Then, *it* happened. My husband became ill – very ill – and I became very, very exhausted. Overnight, I became the sole caretaker for my unwell husband. And, of course, the main caretaker for our four children. My life was suddenly all about giving to everyone else but me: my love, energy, empathy, courage, strength – well, you get my point here ... I gave all of me to all of them. It was like Groundhog Day: another day, but the same routine, the same depletion of energy, the same exhaustion – every single day, until I got to the point where I didn't even know who I was any more. This left me feeling as though I was running on empty. My mood was low, my patience had worn thin and my happiness had been drained.

Where did the high-spirited, energetic, lover of life, ever-happy Julie go? I guess you could say I had hit rock bottom with my own self-care. I had stopped recharging my own batteries, so that I could recharge everyone else's.

I am often asked how I found my way back. It wasn't a one-day fix, or even a one-week or one-month fix. It took a good, solid year of self-care that I still continue to embrace each and every day of my life.

I found that on the very rare occasions that I did take time out to take care of me during this period I was not only happier and healthier, but I was also a better mother, wife and friend. Then, having noticed how these small moments of self-care made me and those around me feel, I realised that I needed to start taking care of myself every single day, not just once in a while. I also realised that I could do this in seemingly small ways – I didn't have to take a whole day or an afternoon to focus on myself. I could do it in a few minutes – anywhere, anytime. And when I did, I felt as though I could take on anything. My energy levels were transformed, my smile reappeared and I was laughing again. I became healthy in body, mind and spirit and, most importantly, perhaps, I was recharged every single day!

Since making an ongoing commitment to my own self-care, I have had the energy I need to power through each day, the patience to be present for everyone who needs me and unlimited enthusiasm and passion for life.

Now I want to help you do the same.

Slowing Down for Self-care

When we nourish ourselves and start to incorporate even the smallest moments of self-care we tap into an energy within us that's always been there, even when we are depleted. This energy is different to the energy that powers us through the day. It allows us to slow down, to listen to our gut instincts and to ourselves.

Making the decision to slow down, instead of finding ways to steam ahead, may seem ridiculous to you. If you have an endless to-do list and demands from countless people then you may think you need to stay in the fast lane. But if you take a moment to slow down, take stock of what is really important to you and then give the lion's share of your energy and attention to those things, you will find you are more fulfilled and less stressed out.

Is Self-care Selfish?

Unfortunately, so many of us (past me included) think of self-care as a 'selfish' act. We see it as something that we do after we've taken care of everyone else, and after we've got everything else done. But let's be honest: when do we really ever get all those tasks on our to-do list done?

Authentic self-care is about nurturing ourselves for our own benefit and that of those around us. Dr Andrew Weil, a guru of alternative medicine and one of my personal heroes, uses the heart as the perfect example of self-care, and I often share this analogy in my yoga class. He explained to American TV and radio host Larry King that, 'Each time the heart beats, it first pumps blood to itself, then to the rest of the body. It has to work this way in order for us to stay alive. The same is true for us human beings. We have to take care of ourselves first, so we can take care of others.'

Self-care isn't about doing anything 'perfectly' or 'right'. It is about taking time out for ourselves, on a daily basis, in order to think better, feel better and move better. When we do that we become more efficient and have *so* much more energy every single day. And we become more compassionate with ourselves and with others.

So, no, self-care is most definitely not selfish.

Different Types of Self-care

I believe that there are two main types of self-care: recreational and transformative. Both are necessary, but they serve different purposes.

Recreational self-care is a quick escape, like a massage, any kind of 'spa' appointment, a weekend getaway or a vacation. This type of self-care lifts our spirits and mood temporarily, clears the mind for a while and allows us to 'let go' in the short term. All of this is, of course, good.

Transformative self-care is on a whole different level, whereby we are able to nourish ourselves deep within and not just on the surface. This kind of self-care is an investment in our present and future well-being and overall happiness. And it's permanent. But we must sacrifice some of our time and energy so that we can truly recharge for life.

I know that recreational self-care feels easier and, well, it is. It is a welcome distraction, an escape and an emotional reprieve, and it can almost numb us from wanting to go deeper into transformative self-care. But I think we all know the easy way is usually not the best way. Yes, transformative self-care will be harder, but it will be worth it, giving us healing, sustained energy, inner growth, confidence, self-love, passion and, ultimately, purpose in life.

Transformative self-care isn't a guilty pleasure. It's actually an important part of your journey towards long-term health and happiness. So at the heart of my plan is you making a commitment to your health, to your happiness, and to *you* – and that takes time. But spending time on you . . . well, that's the beginning of your self-care journey. This book will help, but it starts with you.

There is a saying, 'The longest relationship you have in your life is with yourself'. This perfectly illustrates where you should place yourself on your list of priorities. Over the next twelve months you will learn how to become your own best friend and how to recharge for life. You owe it to yourself – to you: your best friend.

The Plan

We are going to work on a different aspect of self-care each month in order to form real, lasting habits that become a permanent part of everyday life.

Studies have shown that it takes twenty-eight days to create a habit and twenty-eight days to break one. My twelve-month plan will help you develop a new self-care habit each and every month. Oh, and I bet you'll find that you'll also be breaking one or two bad habits along the way, too. And that's OK!

Each month includes some form of recreational self-care which, as I said earlier, we do need. But the bulk of each month is about transformative self-care: taking small moments out of your day to work on you. Each month focuses on different areas of your life to create a well-rounded sense of self instead of simply focusing on one or two aspects of self-care. Here's a little glimpse of the different types of self-care you will be exploring each month.

Month One: Love of food vs love of eating: Eating the right foods mindfully

This month is all about understanding your relationship with food and how you can eat to nourish your body and mind. We will talk about eating the right foods at the right times, and how you can adjust your dietary habits to boost your health.

Month Two: Managing stress

In Month Two, we will look at the prevalence of stress in our society and how it impacts our health and happiness. We'll discuss practical techniques for dealing with stress and work on how we can change how we respond to it.

Month Three: Digital detox

Month Three explores how technology affects our lives, and I will share my tips for limiting use of digital devices in order to stay more connected to the real world.

Month Four: Rebuilding self-esteem and becoming optimistic

Here, we take a look at reasons why your self-esteem may be low and discuss realistic ways to tackle them. Through various techniques, I will show how you can become a much more optimistic and confident person.

Month Five: Alleviating anxiety

In Month Five, we will be working to understand how and why anxiety can become such a huge problem. I will share simple but effective techniques for alleviating anxiety and for lessening its impact on all areas of your life.

Month Six: Finding, believing and building your passions

Month Six is all about finding your passions, beginning to believe in them and building realistic goals around them. I will explain how you can achieve the right mindset for doing this, in addition to sharing other useful tools and techniques.

Month Seven: Shining your authentic light and finding your truth

In Month Seven, we are going to look at what it means to live an authentic and honest life, the endless benefits of doing so, and how we can all shine our lights continuously.

Month Eight: Mastering your inner critic

Month Eight will tackle the difficult topic of the inner critic – the voice inside all of us that tries to keep us down. We will look at how to silence this voice and rewire our minds with positivity instead.

Month Nine: Learning to love yourself
In Month Nine we are going to learn to love ourselves. We will consider the benefits of self-love and how we all can and should accept love and appreciate ourselves for the amazing, unique people that we are.

Month Ten: Say goodbye to fear and hello to courage
Expelling fear from our lives and inviting courage in is the topic for this month. We examine the reasons why fear can be so detrimental to happiness and practical ways in which we can overcome the fears that we each struggle with.

Month Eleven: Live with purpose and permit yourself to change
Here, we will explore how we can live our lives with greater purpose and benefit emotionally from doing so. I want you to see how embracing positive change can help you to create the life for yourself that you truly want.

Month Twelve: Enhance your happiness and spread it around

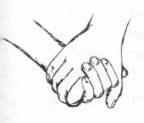

In our final month I will show you how you can enhance your own happiness and benefit from spreading this happiness to those around you.

What to Expect

In each month you'll find a questionnaire to get you thinking, but at the heart of each month's theme are the 'Self-care Actions' – exercises that will help you put all my advice into practice. OK, it's homework, but it won't be scored, judged or critiqued by anyone else, unless you choose to share it. Rather, think of it as an opportunity for you to write from your heart, to feel from your gut, to put it all down on paper, so you can actually see in writing what your inner self – your true, authentic self – is telling you. You can either journal straight into this book in the spaces provided or use your own dedicated notebook as your twelve-month journal.

You will also find some 'Tips to Recharge' – these are things that you can do to help you along the road to self-care. At the back of the book, you will find a bonus 21-day challenge that you can do any time after the twelve-month plan: this comprises twenty-one little self-care nuggets to remind you how easy it is to incorporate self-care into your everyday life. You'll also find some blank pages where you can make extra notes.

You don't need to wait for January to start the plan; you can begin whenever you want, so if you get this book in May, your opening chapter is still 'Month One'. But try to follow the order and not skip months. I've purposely themed and placed them in a particular sequence as each one builds on the previous month.

At first, twelve months might seem like a really long time, but look at it this way: first, a whole year goes by incredibly quickly and second, you get to spend an entire year (not just six weeks or ten days or one quick-fix week) on you! What better cause to devote the next year of your life to than the health, happiness and care of you?

QUESTIONNAIRE: What's your motivation?

Before you turn the page to Month One, take a moment to answer the following questions in your own words and with your own feelings. There is no right or wrong answer. You just need to be honest with yourself. No one else, just you. So go deep inside of you and allow the words to come out authentically and honestly. You will find that being honest with yourself is the first step in committing to embracing self-care and being able to truly recharge.

- Are you recharging for you or for someone else?

- What will you gain if you stick with this twelve-month plan to recharge?

- What will you lose if you incorporate small moments of self-care into your daily life?

- What are the obstacles that have prevented you from taking care of you in the past?

- How much support can you get from others as you attempt to recharge over these next twelve months?

And suddenly you know: it's time to
start something new and trust the
magic of beginnings.

MEISTER ECKHART

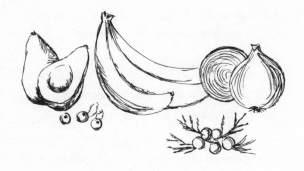

Month One

Eating the Right Foods Mindfully

When you are stressed, you eat ice cream, cake,
chocolate and sweets. Why? Because stressed
spelled backwards is desserts.

ANONYMOUS

The first month is all about the love of food versus the love of eating. The connection between our love of food and our consumption of it is the driver of many of today's health problems. We tend to equate volume with value, quantity with quality, and love or celebrations with overeating.

We may claim to love food but, think about it, are we really savouring it? Notice people when they eat, and well, it's a bit of a panic, and in five minutes the meal is over. Eating becomes a chore. Instead of sitting at the table to enjoy our meals, we tend to distract ourselves with the television, or by talking on the phone while we eat.

When I was younger, I lived on junk food. Everything I ate was highly processed and came in a packet or a jar. At the time, I didn't even know what highly processed meant – I just thought food was food, regardless of how it was made and where it came from. I ate like that for many years, never looking at labels because if it was sold in my local supermarket, then surely it was OK. And the same went for eating out. Again, fast-food outlets had to be OK because they were in my nearest shopping centre. But, as we all now know, processed and packaged 'junk' foods are detrimental to our health. However, it is so easy to binge or 'stuff down' our emotions with these types of food because they taste so good. And so we just keep going back for more.

My Love Affair with Real Food

My love affair with real food began when my husband was ill. I wanted to cure him, but I'm no doctor so food was my way of helping with his recovery. But I wanted to cure me too! While I wasn't technically 'ill', I was depleted of energy and my moods would fluctuate wildly from being upset, angry and sad to being reasonably OK.

I am also the first to hold my hands up and admit to many nights of emotional binge eating. Taking care of everyone else took its toll on me, and I can't even begin to count the number of times I opened my fridge, glared at its contents, pulled something out (it didn't really matter what it was) and just ate and ate and ate – all because I was an emotional wreck. I was eating to fill a void; to try to hide my despair. I wasn't eating for energy, for nutrition or as a way to heal my body. I was actually doing the opposite. I was hurting my body which, ultimately, was hurting me.

I'd always known the famous Hippocrates quote, 'Let food be thy medicine and medicine be thy food', but I had never really tried to understand what it meant until this period in my life. After reading up on how food can affect both mood and energy levels, the penny finally dropped and I started making changes. I wanted to further my knowledge and completed a selection of online nutrition courses, which helped me to get really clear on exactly which foods are great for our health, and exactly how they can help. I soon discovered, for example, how antioxidants can combat the presence of stress hormones in the body and how certain carbohydrates can increase levels of serotonin – the happy hormone.

I bought every nutrition book out there, but I stayed away from dieting books. I wanted to learn about food – real food – and what it could do for my body, mind and spirit. I wasn't interested in calorie counting or faddy diets.

So was Hippocrates right? Can food be medicine? My research into food and experimenting with it convinced me that yes, it *can* heal. And not just physically, but mentally and emotionally. When we choose to nourish our bodies with the vitamins, minerals and other nutrients that it is crying out for, then we can heal, we can be healthy and we can be recharged.

Finding the Right Foods For You

You more than likely know which foods are wrong for you – those high-calorie treats or excessively sugary snacks that leave you feeling lethargic or always craving more. But do you know which foods are right for your body?

Unfortunately, it isn't always as simple as labelling certain foods as good and others as bad. This is because as people, we are all unique, and the things that we need vary from person to person. For example, you may be an athlete who needs to consume a specific number of calories to perform at your peak, or you might be a mother of two and need to eat to energise your body and keep your mind balanced. But there are some basic principles that everyone can benefit from.

The key to choosing the right foods for your body is to avoid anything that has been pre-prepared and comes in plastic packaging, ready to be heated in the microwave. Junk food, fast food – whatever you want to call it – is not going to do your body or your mind any good. Instead, you need to discover which foods leave you feeling satiated and full of energy – these are likely to be plant-based wholefoods that are bursting with feel-good nutrients.

Emotional Eating

Emotional eating is the act of using food to temporarily make ourselves feel better, as opposed to eating because our body tells us it's hungry. Many of us turn to food to relieve stress or boredom, or to comfort us when we need a friend. But what happens when we eat like this? Well, we often begin to feel even worse and the emotions that we've been trying to hide or cover up or even get rid of remain. And worse, they may now be accompanied by another negative emotion – guilt.

So in Month One, we are going to learn to understand the difference between being physically and emotionally hungry. Once we have established that, we are going to look at the emotional triggers that cause us to open that fridge and grab anything. We are on a mission to find other ways to deal with stress, boredom, loneliness or anxiety. And finally, to learn how to just step back and pause before giving in to emotional eating.

Understanding emotional eating

For many people, eating is their main emotional coping mechanism (that's why we are addressing it in the first month). I'm not saying that from time to time when we use food to celebrate or to reward ourselves, or even as a pick-me-up, that it's necessarily a bad thing. But we do need to recognise why we are eating certain things, and then start to gain power over the foods we eat and our feelings, rather than the other way around. So start by answering some questions. Grab your journal or simply write your answers here:

QUESTIONNAIRE: Are you an emotional eater?

- Does your appetite increase when you are stressed?

- Does food comfort you in a similar way to having a companion?

- Do you often continue eating when you know that you are already full?

- Do you use food to reward yourself?

- Do you eat when you are experiencing negative feelings, such as sadness or anxiety?

- Do you feel you have little power over your dietary habits?

Answering these questions will help you recognise how prone you are to emotional eating. Let's go a bit deeper now to find out a bit more about what triggers us to eat emotionally.

Emotional versus physical hunger

Understanding the difference between emotional and physical hunger makes it much easier to distinguish between the two. When we are physically hungry, the hunger comes on slowly. Think about the times when you felt a bit hungry and then, as time went on, you felt more and more hungry until you thought, 'OK, I need to eat!' This is physical hunger. But with emotional hunger, you feel you need to eat right now, as though it's a matter of urgency.

When you are physically hungry, your stomach growls and you feel as if anything will satisfy you – even vegetables! When you are emotionally hungry, however, you crave something in particular – a pizza, a tub of ice cream, an entire bag of crisps – and nothing else will do. This, in turn, leads to mindless eating – you don't really enjoy what you're eating, you just 'need' to eat it.

When you are physically hungry, you eat until you are full, not stuffed. Emotional eating, on the other hand, is about eating until you are uncomfortably stuffed. (I have many memories of having to unbutton my jeans without being seen to do so!)

But I think the biggest distinction between emotional and physical hunger is this: when you are emotionally hungry, the hunger pain isn't located in the stomach as it is when you are physically hungry. Emotional hunger is located in your head – you can't get the craving, the food, the emotion out of your mind.

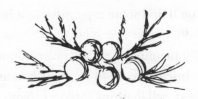

Causes of emotional eating

Emotional eating is linked to our feelings, but situations, places and even people can cause it too. I'm sure you can think of a time when you didn't feel great – maybe you felt uncomfortable, insecure or uneasy – and you used food to help you 'get through' that situation or 'deal' with that person. At these times, and when these feelings arise, we need to identify our emotional eating triggers.

First on that list is stress. Stress can make you emotionally hungry. And, in our fast-paced world, with the demands of home and work life, high levels of the stress hormone cortisol can be a serious problem. Cortisol is released by the adrenal glands (small glands situated on top of the kidneys) and, when we have too much of it in our bloodstreams, we experience cravings for junk foods, salty and sweet foods, fried foods and processed and packaged foods – the foods that give us that instant, but short-lived burst of energy. This, ultimately, is a form of pleasure eating.

The more stress there is in your life, the more likely you are to eat emotionally, unless you find ways to control these urges – distracting yourself with an activity, for example. (You'll find some suggestions on how to do this on pages 27–9).

As I briefly mentioned earlier on, emotional eating is also a way to briefly silence feelings, such as anger, shame, guilt, loneliness, self-loathing, anxiety, pain, sadness and even resentment. Even boredom or a feeling that we have no purpose can be a trigger, and so we emotionally eat because we are dissatisfied with life. By numbing ourselves with food, we feel we can numb our feelings.

Foods we were given as children can have emotional connections, too. Perhaps you were given food when you did something good or when you were feeling sad? Or perhaps your emotional eating is driven by the nostalgia of childhood memories, such as your mum's signature home-made lasagne. Getting together for social occasions with family or friends can certainly lead to emotional overeating: everyone else is eating, the food is flowing and those around you encourage you to keep eating – try this, have that, eat one of those. Some social situations can also make us nervous, and what do we do when we're nervous? We eat!

Recognising emotional-eating triggers
Answer the following questions about how you feel when you emotionally eat.

QUESTIONNAIRE: What are your triggers?

- Are you angry with yourself or someone else?

- Do you feel you're not good enough?

- Do you feel stressed?

- Are you feeling pain?

- Do you struggle to feel good about yourself through-out your day?

- Do you feel that your life is super-tough and unfair compared to others?

When we start to recognise our emotions right away, we can grasp when we are eating as a way of coping. But let's be honest, stopping ourselves can be very difficult. Having said that, we can be much more powerful over our food cravings than we give ourselves credit for.

Just because you have tried to resist emotional eating in the past and might have failed doesn't mean that you aren't powerful enough to try again. You just need to find healthy alternatives to food that you can turn to in order to feel fulfilled.

ACCEPT YOUR FEELINGS

It's important to acknowledge that whatever feelings you have before you grab that tub of ice cream, biscuit or chocolate bar are valid. You are entitled to your feelings and now you need to either sort out the situation or simply accept that right now you're not feeling great inside. Understand that we learn from everything, every situation, every person, every feeling. I like to think of it as an opportunity to grow.

SELF-CARE ACTION: Combat emotional eating

When the urge to eat emotionally appears, try doing one of the following instead:

- Record your thoughts about your food urges in a journal.
- Come up with your own powerful mantra. For

example: 'I won't let these feelings consume me and therefore, I won't emotionally eat!'

- Take a five-minute walk. Even if you're at work – walk around the office or around the block.
- Hug your partner, your friend, your kids or your pets – this releases oxytocin, the 'love hormone', and that makes you feel better.
- Take five minutes to look through photos of yourself with friends. Photos from a holiday or from times that make you smile are often best!
- List three things you like about yourself and stick the list on your fridge.
- Remind yourself of when you coped well in a situation or with your feelings: you've done it before, so you can do it again.
- Call the person who always makes you feel better.
- Put some calming music on and drink a cup of tea.
- Pick up this book and read this chapter again.

There are also certain practical steps you can take to make it less likely that the urge will appear in the first place:

- Throw out the unhealthy foods that you already have in your kitchen and commit to not buying any more when you go grocery shopping. By removing temptation, you are less likely to experience those urges.
- Remember, emotional eating is virtually a mindless

act and you are pretty much on autopilot when it happens. Before you know it, you've reached for that bag of crisps or sweets, and they're gone in a flash. But what if you just paused for five minutes? That's my challenge to you: take a look at the food on your fork or in your hand before you put it in your mouth. If that mouthful is going to do more harm than good, make the choice to love yourself instead with a healthier option. And make a conscious effort to appreciate every mouthful. This will help to adjust your thinking when it comes to eating. Everything that you put into your body should serve to nourish you in some way.

Mindfulness and Emotional Eating

When we eat emotionally, we don't feel strong enough to deal with our feelings head-on, so we try to avoid them by eating food. Allowing ourselves to actually feel our emotions can be scary. But, by learning to just *be* with our feelings – to feel and accept them, rather than suppress them – we learn to become mindful. And this mindfulness can then extend to our eating habits.

Mindful eating is a practice that helps us to understand our eating habits, and to develop the five-minute pause between what it was that triggered our emotions (the situation, that person, that thing) and our actions (to eat or not to eat).

Mindful eating has really helped me with my emotional eating. Mindfulness has also really helped me to see, smell, taste and chew my food more. Adopting a mindful eating practice means you truly pay attention to what you're putting into your mouth. In doing so, you become fully attentive and appreciative of your food as you shop for it, cook it, serve it and finally eat it, as you'll see . . .

Shopping For Success

I want you to change the way you think about food, as doing so will set you up for a lifetime of healthy eating. Let's start with your shopping list. I totally get that most of us either go to the supermarket or get online and just buy. We don't necessarily have set recipes in mind when we shop. What I have learned to do is:

- Buy a wide range of wholefoods – for example, fresh vegetables and fruit, whole grains, pulses, nuts and seeds, fresh fish and high quality meat.
- Leave processed and packaged foods out of the basket.
- Steer clear of anything that has more than seven ingredients on the label.
- Shop soon after eating a meal (then there's no temptation to buy anything bad because your body is happy and nourished, and so is more likely to make happier, healthier choices).

Creating Healthy Cooking Habits

You don't have to have set recipes in mind when you are grocery shopping – I rarely do. I just buy the good stuff, bring it home and then have fun creating something terrific. There are plenty of wonderful, wholesome recipes online if you look for them.

Let's say, for example, you've bought a gorgeous aubergine, but aren't sure what to do with it. Search online for aubergine recipes and then be inspired by all that you discover. You can usually morph any recipe into something that you like. Don't be put off if you don't have the exact ingredients that the recipe calls for. If it says to use pine nuts and you only have almonds, use almonds. If it says use quinoa and you have brown rice, use the brown rice. It is super-simple and, personally, I find it much more satisfying to give recipes my own twist.

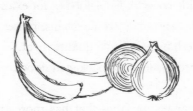

Eating Mindfully

Let's go back to mindful eating for a moment and look at it in more detail. Once you have made your meal, start with a small portion and pause for a couple of minutes before you begin eating. During these moments be grateful for the food on your plate and, if you are sharing the meal with others, be grateful for their company.

As you start to eat your food take small bites so that you can completely taste the food in your mouth. Bring all of your senses to your plate: what do you see, what can you smell, what do you hear when you chew, what are the different textures and tastes? Try to notice all the ingredients, including any seasonings you used.

While you are chewing, set your utensils down in between bites. Chew your food thoroughly enough to really taste it. I try to chew each mouthful between fifteen and twenty times. As well as being more mindful, this also has the added benefit of helping your digestion. The saliva in the mouth might be 98 per cent water, but it's 2 per cent digestive enzymes, which help to break down food before it reaches the stomach. This is advantageous because the biggest strain on our bodies – the internal process that depletes the most energy – is digestion. So by helping our digestion by chewing more, we reserve more energy for after our meal.

Eat slowly. Devote twenty minutes at least to eating your main meal. Not only will this stop you from gorging on your food, but it gives you, your body and your mind a chance to slow down. To just be.

Eat sitting down. (And oh, by the way, eating in your car does not count.) Eat in a calm environment without distractions such as television, radio, reading the newspaper or magazines or intense or difficult conversations.

Eat only what your body wants and not what your head is telling you to eat. Eat with pleasure and eat until you are satisfied, not until you are stuffed. I swear by this rule: eat until you are 80 per cent full.

These simple guidelines are so effective at helping us practice mindful eating and get out of the bad habit of emotional eating. If you find it difficult, don't lose heart – remind yourself that it takes time to develop a healthy habit (see box, below).

BREAK THE HABIT

Remember I said earlier that it takes twenty-eight days to create a habit and twenty-eight days to break one? So can you put off that emotional eating for five minutes? Just put a timer on and wait. And while you're waiting, try one of the actions on pages 27–8, being sure to check in with yourself as you do so: think about how and what you are feeling. What emotions are you experiencing? Then, even if you do end up eating, you'll understand a bit more about why you did it, which will definitely be helpful the next time you get that craving. And I bet you'll have a different response next time around.

In Month One really focus on your feelings, your eating when you have those feelings, the foods you shop for and how you eat your food. Use the tips that I have just shared to create healthy habits and they will soon become second nature – for the rest of your life.

Month Two

Managing Stress

Dear Stress, Let's break up.

Stress, stress, stress. It is probably one of the most often heard words in our modern world – but it is also one of the most dangerous toxins in our lives, as it is implicated in numerous illnesses. In fact, a Harvard study in 2015 suggested that stress is as detrimental to our health as breathing in second-hand smoke. As a society, we have come to believe that being stressed, anxious, angry and down is the norm. But just because stress is common, it doesn't mean that we should simply accept it without attempting to address or resolve the sources of our stress.

The Stress Epidemic

Stress is an epidemic that most of us ignore because we think it's 'normal'. And it's not just our ever-growing to-do lists or our jobs that cause us to feel stressed – it can come from our past, our relationships, our family and yes, even world affairs.

I often used to feel stress physically in my body, with my shoulders becoming super-tight, to the point that they were painful even when I was resting. And I knew it was because I've always tried to do too much too quickly – all of the time. I'd think that if I kept working, kept doing, kept pushing, kept going, then I would finally get everything done. But the reality is that there is never a 'done'. There will always be 'something', and the stress comes from thinking that we still have to do that something. If, like me, you find yourself consumed with stress, welcome to the club! It can appear to those around us that we have it all sorted, but I bet most of us are crying out on the inside, begging to take a break. So this month, let's break up with stress – once and for all.

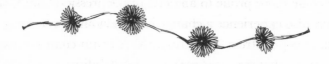

How the Body Reacts to Stress

Before we begin to learn how to manage stress over this next month, let's first try to understand what it does to our bodies, minds and spirits. And trust me, it's not pretty.

Believe it or not, your body does not know the difference between being chased by a sabretooth tiger and having a stressful journey to work, an argument at home or a difficult discussion with your boss, for example. And it can therefore enter fight/flight/freeze mode – basically the body's instinctive mechanism for survival – whether you're being chased by a tiger or panicking about your unrealistic to-do list.

The result is that it produces high levels of the stress hormones cortisol and adrenaline in an attempt to help you cope with what it perceives to be a threat. However, chronic high levels of these hormones in the body negatively impact your health and happiness.

Stress and mental health

Your mental health is likely to suffer first when you are exposed to frequent high levels of stress. You could become more prone to anxiety and depression, and you may also experience a change in behaviour as you struggle to cope. Stress can actually alter brain connectivity, meaning that reactions to fear and the ability to stay calm can be impacted in a detrimental way. And of course it's a vicious circle – experiencing anxiety and depression or other associated mental-health issues can cause further stress – and one that can be extremely difficult to break out of.

Stress and weight

Stress can also affect your weight in an unhealthy way. It increases cravings and emotional eating, as discussed in Month One, and it can slow down the metabolism. This is largely thanks to the increased presence of cortisol when you are stressed out – more cortisol leads to higher insulin levels and lower blood sugar, which can prompt cravings for fatty, sugary foods. At the other end of the spectrum, stress can also make some people lose their appetite, meaning the body doesn't get the nutrients it needs.

Stress and the immune system

When we are stressed, our immune system doesn't work as well – it's stressed out too – so we are more likely to catch that cold or flu that's going around.

The gut is home to the majority of our immune cells, so it's hardly surprising that when we are stressed we are more likely to get ill but also to suffer from gastro-intestinal conditions. The gut is known as the second brain. The entire digestive tract is lined with nervous system neurons, and the responses from these cells are carried up to the brain. Also, the gut contains a massive 95 per cent of your serotonin. Serotonin is your 'happy' neurotransmitter. I, for one, want to be happy, so it pays to look after our gut.

As well as compromising immunity and gastrointestinal disorders, stress is associated with insomnia. I could go on, but I think you get my point: stress makes the body, mind and spirit incredibly unhappy. On a positive note, this is where small moments of self-care can have a huge impact.

QUESTIONNAIRE: How do you deal with stress?

When you have had a stressful, not-so-great kind of a day, what's the first thing that you do?

a) Eat something unhealthy (aka junk food, processed food – you know the kind of food I'm talking about) and sit on the sofa and sulk, watch mind-numbing TV or look on social media and see how 'perfect' everyone else's life is?
b) Go out for a brisk walk, run, yoga – or some other form of exercise?
c) Meditate?
d) Read an inspiring book?
e) Take a candlelit bath?
f) Journal?

If we were being honest, most of us would probably choose answer a). But I want you to go a bit deeper and

find out how stressed out you *really* are by answering the
following questions (I promise you, this little quiz is not
meant to stress you out!).

Tick the answers that are true for you.

1. I don't like to socialise with people, especially when
   I 'have' to.
2. I absolutely dread going back to work after the
   weekend.
3. I dread having to listen to other people's problems – I have no sympathy for them.
4. I don't like to engage in conversation. I like to keep
   it short and simple.
5. Healthy activities like exercise and eating well
   aren't a priority.
6. I feel exhausted and/or have low energy most of
   the time.
7. My to-do list keeps growing and growing.
8. My life feels very claustrophobic.
9. I don't have that much fun any more.
10. I can't push myself to do what I know will make
    me feel better. I feel stuck.

What does this questionnaire tell you? Well, it's simple.
The more answers that you ticked, the more stressed
you are. Of course, we would all like to de-stress (and
I'm going to show you how to do that throughout this

month), because, at the end of the day, we all want to wake up feeling refreshed, alive, happy and ready to take on the day.

Understanding and Managing Stress

The negative effects of stress start to develop when you have more pressure put on you than you are able to handle. It's important to note that this pressure can come from yourself as well as from external sources.

How many times have you mentally said to yourself or to others, 'I'm so stressed out'. Yet stress isn't something that happens *to us*, it happens *inside us*, and the more we remind ourselves that we are stressed out, the more our bodies, minds and spirits are going to think it, feel it and react to it.

Did you know that around 75 per cent of all visits to doctors in the US are for stress-related issues? However, only 3 per cent of those patients actually receive some type of stress-management counselling. This is why Month Two is so important for you and your health.

On my own journey to slow everything down I started to look at my diet and the foods that actually *do* help us to de-stress. Yes, what we eat can do wonders for our stress levels.

Tips to Recharge: Eating to Relieve Stress

Food works to help you feel good from the inside out. Your body loves it when you eat well, as this is when it becomes balanced, your hormone and blood-sugar levels are restored and your body, in general, is happier. During times of stress you need to nourish your body and avoid foods that cause the release of more adrenaline and cortisol, which will only make your body think it needs more energy. Energy for the body comes in the form of food, so naturally you will then feel hungrier and eat more. But it's unlikely to be the food that the body really needs or wants.

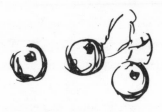

With cortisol floating around the bloodstream, you are encouraging yourself to make poor food choices. Also, the more cortisol there is in the body, the more fat storage occurs, which then leads to weight gain and related health issues. But the good news is that there are foods that help with stress, so the next time you are stressed, make sure you include them in your diet.

Vitamin C

Eat (don't supplement) vitamin C. As you now know, the adrenal glands are nestled on top of the kidneys, and they are in charge of our stress hormones – cortisol and adrenaline. Vitamin C is stored in high concentrations in the adrenal glands. When we are super-stressed, we burn through vitamin C like crazy. So, we want to eat foods that are very high in vitamin C to help us replace it, so that our adrenal glands can function at their optimal level. These include:

- Brussels sprouts
- papaya
- cauliflower
- broccoli
- red peppers
- strawberries
- oranges

Magnesium

Magnesium can help us to relax which, in turn, helps us to de-stress. It is an important mineral for our adrenal glands, and when we are stressed we can actually lose magnesium. This then leads to additional stress and some tight, achy muscles. Foods that are high in magnesium include:

- spinach
- kale
- romaine lettuce

- watercress
- parsley
- coriander

When you eat these greens, you get an extra bonus for your adrenals because dark leafy greens also contain vitamin C.

Gluten-free grains
Fill your pantry with gluten-free grains. Why? Because gluten-free grains are high in B vitamins, which are extremely important for fighting stress. This is because they support the nervous system and brain function. Also, grains are a complex carbohydrate and these carbs can help the brain produce serotonin, that feel-good chemical – what a bonus! Stock up on:

- oats
- quinoa
- brown rice
- buckwheat

Potassium
Potassium is great for keeping stress levels down. This is because it helps to regulate your blood pressure and relaxes your muscles. Potassium is used by every single cell in your body, so when levels are low, you are less able to cope with stress. Foods high in potassium include:

- bananas
- avocados
- citrus fruits
- citrus juices

Before we move on to other stress-busting actions, the following questionnaire will help you identify how you can increase your intake of those all-important stress-busting foods.

QUESTIONNAIRE: Can you improve your anti-stress diet?

1. What vitamin-C-rich foods do you already include in your daily diet and which new ones can you start to incorporate into your diet this month?

2. What magnesium-rich foods do you already include in your daily diet and which new ones can you start to incorporate into your diet this month?

3. What gluten-free grains do you already include in your daily diet and which new ones can you start to incorporate into your diet this month?

4. What potassium-rich foods do you already include
    in your daily diet and which new ones can you start
    to incorporate into your diet this month?

We've now looked at the stress-reducing foods you need to include in your diet at all times. But there's so much more you can do this month to ensure that you are equipped with plenty of stress-fighting tools.

Strategies for Relieving Stress

Besides food, there are other areas we can target to help train our bodies and minds to handle stress in a productive, healthy and mindful way. Once you have acquired these tools, you can whip them out at the first sign of stress, so that you are better equipped to control your stress level before it gets too high.

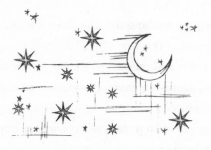

Repeat positive affirmations

The more you hear something – a message, a saying, a quote – the more likely you are to not only remember it, but to believe it too. This is true when we hear messages from our parents, our spouse, our partner, friends, co-workers, bosses and yes, even ourselves. (Side note: don't worry about that just yet – we will be focusing on how to master our own inner critic in Month Eight.)

We can absolutely choose what we want to believe by counteracting negative messages. Trust me, the more we repeat positive affirmations, the more positive, healthy habits we create. And, with time, we can actually rewire our brains to hear the positive more than the negative.

Choose four positive affirmations this month – that's one per week – and repeat them to yourself daily, *especially* in those moments when you encounter a stressful situation. Here are some good ones that have helped me for many years:

- I can handle anything that life throws at me.
- I am at peace, even when life gets crazy.
- Staying calm and relaxed will make me healthier.
- I am transforming into someone who stays cool under pressure.
- Relieving stress on a daily basis is super-important to my well-being.
- Others are noticing how calm and collected I am.

- Being at peace, my life feels more balanced.
- I am starting to live a more balanced life.
- I do at least one small moment of self-care each day to relieve my stress.
- Setbacks will only make me stronger.

SELF-CARE ACTION: My affirmations

Write down your four stress-relieving affirmations here:

Walk outdoors more

Did you know that too much intense physical exercise puts your body under stress? I know that sounds crazy, but it's true. Excess exercise can cause our adrenals to release more cortisol, which is not what we want when we are already stressed out. So during times of stress, it helps simply to take a walk.

Walking outdoors allows us to feel peaceful, giving us much more mental clarity than when we have to think about an exercise routine. It is one of a very few forms of exercise that calm us down. Plus, walking is free, it's easily accessible (it's right outside our front doors) and it doesn't call for special exercise gear. We just have to train our bodies to know that when we are stressed, we should go for a walk. Even if it's raining, snowing or sleeting, we should bundle up and get outside for at least twenty minutes a day.

The benefit of walking outside, as opposed to on the treadmill in the gym, is that you will begin to feel connected to nature, and the fresh air will invigorate and refresh you.

Need some suggestions for getting into walking? My kids know that whenever I have to park the car – whether at the supermarket, the cinema, the shops or workplace – I'll always choose the parking spot farthest away from where we need to be, so that we can then walk to where we need to go. You can also adopt the idea of an after-lunch stroll. No matter where you have lunch – in the office, a restaurant or at home – make it a priority to get outside and walk for twenty minutes afterwards.

Getting outside every single day is a game changer. Oh, and of course there is an added bonus: walking can help to improve digestion and sleep too.

SELF-CARE ACTION: My walking schedule

Ask yourself where in your busy and chaotic day you can incorporate twenty minutes of walking, so that it becomes a habit. Might it be walking to work, to the gym, after breakfast, walking the kids to school, after lunch, during an afternoon break . . .? Figure it out and write it down here:

I will walk:

Making 'Good' Sleep a Priority

I have heard it said that we should be asleep for one third of our lives. If that's the case, we should aim for between seven and eight hours each night (although I appreciate that some people – myself included – need a little less). Sleeping is when our minds and our bodies are finally at ease. And when we allow our bodies to come into the rest-and-digest mode (when we are governed by our parasympathetic nervous system), we give our bodies a break from having probably been in the fight/flight/freeze mode (when our sympathetic nervous system is in charge). If that's just made you think *What?*! bear with me: essentially, the parasympathetic system keeps us in a physical state of balance and a calm state of mind, whereas the sympathetic nervous system keeps us ready and waiting to respond to danger.

Unfortunately, getting a good night's sleep isn't as simple as deciding to go to bed at the right time. If you have had a stressful day, you need to prepare your body for sleep. You can't just go from one hundred to zero in a minute.

You need to educate your body and mind that it's time for sleep – in other words, establish a bedtime routine.

I have had the same bedtime routine for at least five years now, doing literally the same thing every night, even when I'm travelling and not in my own home.

Between thirty and forty-five minutes before bed, I turn off all of my electronic devices. The day is done, as far as I am concerned, and if someone is emailing me this late at night, then it can wait (and they probably need to learn how to de-stress too!). I run a bath and pour in some Epsom salts, then I turn off the lights and light three candles. Epsom salts are high in magnesium, which is absorbed by my body as I soak; and, as my magnesium levels are replenished, I begin to feel calm and relaxed. In the semi-darkened bathroom, I'm telling my body that night has come, and it's time to rest and recharge my batteries overnight. This is how I unwind each and every night without fail.

SELF-CARE ACTION: Bedtime routine

What can you incorporate into your bedtime routine? List your ideas here.

Breathing and Visualisation

Breathing is free, but we often forget about it. We are also prone to restricting our breath and not breathing properly, especially when we are stressed. Yet our breath has the ability to make a difference to our stress levels almost immediately. And it's available to us every single second of every single day.

Studies have shown that breathing for the body (rather than the body breathing for us) is among the most effective ways to calm the central nervous system and bring us back into the rest-and-digest mode described earlier, rather than constantly being in fight/flight/freeze mode.

Many of us will have been told by someone at some point to 'just breathe'. If this applies to you, and you heeded this advice – if only for a moment or two – I suspect you probably noticed that you did feel a little bit better. The truth is that when we are under stress, we tend to hold our breath or breathe short, shallow breaths without even realising.

By creating a conscious practice of focusing on the breath, it virtually becomes our superhero power. It has an almost immediate effect on the heart, lungs and head, resulting in a more balanced mind–body connection, often meaning the difference between a highly charged emotional response and a calm one.

I like to think of the breath as massaging all of your cells, organs and muscles with oxygen. It's like a free stress-busting massage. So when you find yourself feeling stressed, try to either immediately stop what you're doing and breathe *or* breathe through it.

Here is a great breathing exercise. I use it at least five times a day, especially when I'm cycling to and from places. It can be done anywhere, anytime, even in the midst of a stressful conversation, situation or meeting.

SELF-CARE ACTION: Calming breath

- As you start to inhale, breathe in through the nose for a count of four.
- Hold the breath at the top of the lungs for one to two seconds, then exhale out of the nose for five to six seconds.
- Visualise the breath coming in through the nose, down the throat, into the chest, around the heart and ending deep in the belly.
- Pause and hold the breath for one to two seconds, then exhale out of the belly, up to the heart, into the chest, through the throat and out of the nose.

You needn't do this for long periods of time to get the benefits. Even three full breaths in and out of the nose can – and will – help. If you are in the middle of something stressful, try to use this breathing technique throughout the entire situation – in the moment – until the stressful period has ended. Not only will you find that your mind becomes clearer, and that you create more space between each thought, but also that your heart rate slows down. And I bet you'll leave that stressful situation feeling pretty darned good, regardless!

There is also an add-on to this exercise. It's called visualisation – an incredibly powerful technique and one that I swear by each and every day.

When you are in the throes of stress, begin the aforementioned breathing exercise and simply visualise the way you would like to feel at that moment, be it happy, calm, loved, compassionate, empathetic, sympathetic, confident . . .

As you visualise a calmer you, and a happier you, you will literally start to feel your body and mind moving into that mood. Visualising will change your state – mental, physical, emotional – so that you can start feeling the good feelings you would rather have instead!

The simple yet effective strategies listed above should help you to decrease stress the natural way. Every day this month, in order to de-stress, try incorporating these habits into your daily routine. I am confident that by the end of the month you will be feeling much more peaceful.

Other Tips for Tackling Stress

In addition to the above techniques and strategies, there are other ways in which to adjust your mindset and work to embrace a more positive attitude. And, in the process, your mind will become a place in which it is difficult for stress to thrive.

First, stop being so hard on yourself – we will learn about mastering your inner critic in Month Eight, but acknowledging that self-judgement gets you nowhere, and that it ultimately just causes more stress, is beneficial this month, too.

Second, accept that all of your feelings are valid and give yourself the freedom to express them. Don't let them stay in your head. Remember that what others think of you is not your problem; you can't control them or their feelings. And if you are struggling to express your feelings, then simply laugh! Laughter is a great way to relieve stress and to distract the mind.

Try to incorporate all of these small moments of self-care into your daily life over the course of the next month. Then go back to the quiz on page 40 and retake it, comparing how you felt at the start of the month with how you feel after a month of stress-busting.

As you progress with lowering your exposure to stress and better managing your responses to stressful situations, you can expect your mental health to become more balanced and your happiness to shine through. You will also notice that you place less importance on getting through your to-do list, opening yourself up to the possibilities of mindfulness – such as a more relaxed and peaceful frame of mind.

Month Three

Digital Detox

Sometimes you just have to unplug from
everything to find yourself again.

ROBIN LEE

The definition of detoxing is 'to abstain from or rid the body of toxic or unhealthy substances'. The word 'detox' in association with diet has had a bad rap recently. It used to be *the* thing to do, but it's actually not cool anymore to starve yourself of certain things. Our bodies are clever and they will detox themselves without having to deprive ourselves of food, or go on a ten-day juice cleanse.

While a diet detox isn't the way to go, we can most definitely benefit from a digital detox. OK, I know that a month without all of our digital gadgets probably isn't feasible for most of us – we work, we have families, people need to communicate with us and vice versa. But hear me out. What we are aiming for is to stay plugged in while at the same time digitally detoxing. This will help us to feel more at peace but, crucially, feeling more connected to the things that actually make us happy and fulfilled.

You may be someone who is always talking on the phone, but who isn't that interested in checking out Facebook every five minutes. Or you may be an avid social-media user, but rarely use your digital devices for verbal communication. When it comes to a digital detox, we will all have different goals, but each of us can benefit from it in similar ways. So use the advice in this chapter to devise your own individual goals and achieve the best outcomes for you.

The Dangers of Digital

There is growing evidence that too much exposure to digital devices could actually be harming us physically, mentally and emotionally. For example, the constant tapping of your screen could give you a strained neck and back, while the heat from mobile phones just might be penetrating your brain. Plus, the volume on your phone, when placed to your ear, could impair your hearing, and your Wi-Fi signal could be adversely affecting your sleep.

The digital world is not all bad obviously and there are some fantastic benefits. However, in this digital age we need to learn how to keep our physical bodies healthy, our minds sound and our emotions intact. I mean, let's be honest, look around you – in your home – and you'll see digital devices everywhere: on the worktops, on the walls, in your hands, in your children's/partner's/roommate's hands. We have become slightly (if not seriously) addicted to technology. And addiction of any sort is not a good thing.

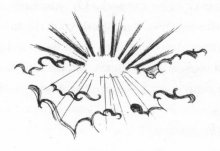

Regaining Control

We need to learn how to put the devices down, put them away – and know that we are OK without them from time to time. We need to be in control of our technology and not the other way around.

This month is all about establishing a healthy relationship with our digital devices. When we are constantly looking at our Instagram feed, refreshing Facebook, checking our emails or newsfeeds, often for no reason at all, then we lose the opportunity to take care of ourselves. We lose the available time for those small moments of self-care.

Now, what's more important? Idly checking your phone

all day or detaching from technology for a few moments to tap into your interests, your hobbies and yourself?

The Mobile Phone

I am sure you have heard that radiation is emitted when you hold your phone to your ear. However, what many people don't realise is that wired headsets do not protect your brain from this radiation. It is far better, therefore, to use your speakerphone button more. So when you get a call – if you can – put it on speakerphone. Your head will thank you.

And what about texting, you ask? A brilliant study in the journal *Surgical Technology International* suggests that when we look down at our devices, the pressure on our neck is equivalent to 60 pounds! When I started to get a really sore neck, I spent a lot of money on massages that really didn't help. But then I did some research and realised my problem was caused by the way I was texting. Once I made sure to keep my neck long and not bent, the pain subsided and both my body and my wallet were happier.

Given that the average amount of time we spend on our mobile phones – according to the app analytics provider Flurry – is two hours and forty-two minutes *every day*, we should all make sure that we keep those necks long when we do look down at our phones.

Another side effect of being glued to our phones is emotional eating (see Month One). Many of us consume junk food while we are on our phones – we eat without thinking about it, snacking on unhealthy foods while staring at our screens. So, be aware of that and stop yourself the next time it happens.

And what about when you are out to dinner with friends or family? Do you place your phone on the table? How about hiding it in your handbag or pocket, turning it on 'mute', so that you can't even hear or feel it. By doing so you'll be making a commitment to giving your friends and family your undivided attention.

Being attached to your phone can also mean that you risk losing much-needed rest. It is so easy to take your phone to bed with you, thinking you will spend just a few minutes catching up on your social-media feeds, then still be staring at it an hour later. In addition, the blue light emitted from your screen can severely disrupt your sleep cycle, so I recommend keeping your phone in a different room and not looking at it in the run-up to bedtime (as per my suggestions on developing a bedtime routine on page 50–1).

Emails

This month is about decluttering and creating more space to breathe, to focus on ourselves, to just be. A good way to start is by clearing out and deleting emails from your inbox and junk folder, as well as messages you have actually never read. Most of us could more likely than not unsubscribe from many of the newsletters that clutter our inboxes. Try to unsubscribe as soon as you get an email from a chain that you never read. Then organise your emails into folders, deleting folders that you no longer use.

I always used to feel the need to respond to emails as soon as possible – especially those that brought out some kind of emotion in me. I remember one in particular that had me super-heated. I was all set to respond right away with a snippy email, but my dad gave me the best advice. He asked if I actually needed to reply immediately, and what would happen if I waited twenty-four hours? The reality was that it wasn't urgent at all; it was just that the email had made me very angry. But that meant I was more likely to respond with anger or with another unhealthy emotion – and what good would that do? So I took my dad's advice and waited for twenty-four hours, after which my response was certainly much more calm and considered than it would have been a day earlier.

As a result, I have developed a healthy habit of taking time – sometimes days – to reply to emails. What's the rush? Ninety-nine per cent of the time there is *no* rush; we just assume that as quickly as emails come into our inbox, we need to get a response back out.

Another good habit to put into practice is to use your automated 'Out of office' facility more often. When you take a lunch break, head to a meeting or are simply away from your digital device, why not put on the out-of-office notification for an hour or two, asking senders to call you if their message is urgent? I bet you won't get one phone call – because, like I said, 99 per cent of the time our emails are not urgent.

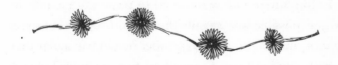

Stressed Out by Technology

Studies have shown that people who use their digital devices the most are also the most stressed out and anxious during their free time. Overuse of these devices, especially when it comes to the internet, can become a serious addiction.

A really good question to ask yourself is, 'Am I checking my devices because I need to respond to something or am I checking them because I have FOMO?' (fear of missing out). If it's the latter, this is a glaring sign that you need to digitally detox throughout your day. If it seems a bit too much to do all of this at the same time, then just commit to changing one habit at a time – perhaps one each week.

One good idea you and your family could perhaps benefit from is 'phone stacking' at mealtimes. It works like this: everyone involved puts their digital device in the middle of the table and the first one to reach for theirs has to clear up at the end of the meal or make the next round of tea or coffee.

Also, if you drive, you will know that it can be tempting to check your device as soon as you hear a ping, even though we all know that doing so while driving is dangerous and illegal. Get into the habit of putting your device in the glove compartment. If you do need to check your phone, pull over safely, check and then put it away again before you carry on. Once you get used to this, you will not only feel safer on the road, but your mind will begin to clear and you can even practise your other new self-care habit: breathing (see page 51)!

SELF-CARE ACTION:
Cutting back and creating time

I want you to list all of your digital devices. Yes, *all* of them, here:

Next, make a list of all the things you really enjoy doing, but aren't doing – you know, your hobbies: tennis, cooking, reading, travelling, drawing – the things you always say you will do later, once you've got through your to-do list.

By cutting back on your digital device usage, you will regain a lot of time – time you can use to do the things that you might actually consider to be more important and more meaningful than constantly checking your phone.

I'll admit, it can be weird at first to 'let go' of your phone and simply be with yourself. But, in order to take better care of yourself, you do need to disconnect from your devices *every single day* .

Ask yourself the following:

- Do you freak out when your phone or other devices are in the 'red' zone for battery supply?
- Do you find ways to conserve your devices' energy to make them last longer (say, switching to 'Do not disturb' mode, lowering the brightness level or closing down apps)?
- Do you have a rechargeable battery pack or plug that you take everywhere with you, so your device never runs out of battery?

Hands up, please!

Now, the next question is: why are we constantly trying to recharge our devices' batteries, rather than our own? Are we not more important than that piece of technology?

Daily Healthy Habits

Technology is ramping up and up, with ever more 'must-have' gadgets available and more screens to look at. That's why it is so important to create daily healthy habits to digitally detox. The idea here is that when this month ends, you will have developed a healthy habit that will be with you for life.

So, to recap on what I've touched upon so far in this chapter, here's a summary of the daily digital detox tips you can use to become healthier and happier, and to really, truly recharge the battery inside of you – not the one in your device!

SELF-CARE ACTION: Taking charge

- Use the speakerphone setting more often.
- Keep your neck long when texting.
- Snack on something healthy rather than unhealthy when on your digital devices.
- Put mobile phones away or on 'Do not disturb' when eating a meal.
- Delete emails that are no longer of use.
- Organise files and documents into folders.
- Wait at least twenty-four hours to respond to emails with emotional triggers.
- Use your 'Out of office' facility more.

Switching Off

We should be switching off all of our devices at certain periods during the day. My rule at home is no digital anything even vaguely in the vicinity at mealtimes: all technology has to be turned off and kept in a separate room to prevent temptation!

How about creating a technology box where all devices go before you sit down to a meal? That way, you can also incorporate what you mastered in Month One in regard to mindful eating. Remember, mindful eating is a form of self-care, and so these non-digital mealtimes give you the perfect opportunity to practise and introduce a small moment of self-care into your everyday life. (If that's a step too far for the moment, try my stacking tip outlined earlier.)

I hope you are starting to see a pattern with the themed months and how they all work together.

Another period of the day when you should switch off is bedtime. When you constantly look at your digital devices before bed, the blue light emitted that I mentioned earlier can have a detrimental effect on your sleep and deplete levels of melatonin. Melatonin is a hormone that induces sleep. It's made by the pineal gland in the brain, but this gland is only activated when it is dark. Generally, melatonin levels will remain elevated during the night, and then dwindle again as it becomes light. So continued exposure to the light from your device as you are winding down can actually hinder your ability to sleep – and to sleep well.

Social Media and Notifications

We lose so much time every day to pointlessly over-checking our social-media feeds and the time has now come to claim it back. When it comes to phones, iPads or anything that 'alerts' or 'notifies' us – turn *off* as many of those push notifications as you can. Personally, I only keep my email notification on. Other than that, all Instagram, Twitter and Facebook alerts are off.

And while you're at it, use this month to purge: purge Facebook groups that you never use any more (even your Facebook 'friends') and unsubscribe from newsletters, sites or blogs that you don't actually read.

Many of us use digital devices when we exercise, so it's very tempting when we are on the treadmill to check when a device vibrates. To avoid that temptation, try to always put your phone on aeroplane mode.

Summary: Tone down the 'noise'

- Switch off all digital devices before bed.
- Turn push notifications *off*.
- Do a social-media purge and unsubscribe.
- Put your phone on aeroplane mode when you're exercising.

Life Beyond Digital Devices

Now that all of your devices are switched off so that you can spend some quality time with you, what do you do?

Before you go to bed at night, it's always nice to take an Epsom-salt, candlelit bath. (Like I said in Month Two, I take one every night before bed and hope you do now, too.) Or you can read a *real* book (like this one!) and not an e-book device that emits blue light. Yes, e-book devices also do that.

Rather than being on your phone during your lunch break, go for a walk to clear your head, if you can. Remember that it's great to walk to help your body digest after eating. If you are eating at home, just take a walk around the block after you have eaten. And don't eat at your desk while catching up on browsing the internet. Leave your screen and get outside in the fresh air, rain or shine – and how about leaving your phone too?

Set aside twenty minutes three times a week to power walk. Put this in your calendar, so you see it as part of your upcoming week. And, if you have to move your walk for whatever reason, don't delete it – just reschedule it! Walk to work and don't check your phone until you arrive. Get your kids ready in the morning and get them to school before checking your phone. Are you noticing a pattern here? We need to get off our digital devices as much as we possibly can!

If you are wondering how to introduce all this into your

day, then why not allocate a set time each day that you will recharge and digitally detox? This can be just ten minutes (or more – even better) every day when you disconnect completely from all things digital and take a moment to just breathe deeply. Regardless of where you are at this time, just close your eyes and visualise something that makes you happy!

SELF-CARE ACTION: Allocating time

Write down the time(s) each day when you are going to digitally detox:

Monday

....

Tuesday

....

Wednesday

....

Thursday

....

Friday

....

Saturday

....

Sunday

....

Team Up to Tackle Stress

If you're still finding all of this quite difficult, try teaming up with someone who can be your digital-detox buddy. I can guarantee that, in this day and age, with the amount that we all have on our plates and the number of devices we own, it won't be hard to find someone to pair up with for a detox. You can then encourage each other to keep going and actually socialise with your buddy for a tea, lunch or dinner to which neither of you brings your digital devices. And tell everyone! The more people you

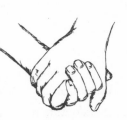

tell, the more people will be impressed with you and the more you will be determined to carry on. Setting an example to friends, family, and your children, especially, is important, so that they will then learn from you.

SELF-CARE ACTION:
Recruit a digital-detox buddy

My digital detox buddy this month is:

Digital detoxing is very much like dieting – there will be cravings. So you need activities to distract you when those cravings – those urges to check your devices – kick in. Go back to the list you made at the beginning of this month of all the things you really enjoy doing, but you aren't doing enough of (see page 64), and do those instead. Doing them will keep you in the present moment. And when you stay in the present moment, you will start to develop a deeper connection with your friends and family, you will truly enjoy that walk outdoors and that healthy meal you made. In short, you will start to feel *recharged*, each and every day.

Kathy's Story

One of my clients, Kathy, digital detoxes before bedtime and whenever the kids are around.

'I decided to do four weeks of digital detox, which meant not being on my mobile phone in the evenings before going to bed and not checking my phone as much as I do when my three kids are around.

'One specific moment with my kids is the school run in the morning and afternoon. We spend forty-five minutes to an hour each morning and afternoon in London traffic jams. I've been doing the same school run for nearly three years now and I ended up being on my mobile phone often (while at a standstill, of course), checking messages, emails and social media. And the same applied to my son, who got his first mobile phone eight months ago. Picture the two of us sitting next to each other, not communicating at all, and my younger two girls – who don't have phones yet – frustrated while I missed things they were telling me.

'So I told my kids I was going to do this four-week detox project and asked my son to do the same. Instead of picking up my phone during these four weeks, I started to ask my kids lots of questions, even when they were not always in the mood to talk. My mission was to push for talks, which was not difficult with my girls, but harder with my eleven-year-old son, who always answered with, 'I am fine', or, 'All good', and that's it. But by making him put his phone down, we slowly came back to having short conversations. In fact, the most amazing thing is that we started to talk more in the evening before going to bed. I took more time to read books to my kids, but the most important thing to me during this period was talking with my son. The more we did it, the more he talked to me and really enjoyed it. It became our evening ritual and now – even though our four-week project has ended – he is the one asking me to come and talk to him about his day, his feelings, his friends and about my day too. I found that getting off my phone really changed my perspective. It made me think more about the things in my life that really matter and, at the end of each day, I definitely feel more recharged.'

Month Four

Rebuilding Your Self-Esteem and Becoming Optimistic

Low self-esteem is like driving through
life with your handbrake on.

MAXWELL MALTZ

Who actually am I? This is one of the biggest questions I asked myself in the past – over and over again, whether in the midst of tears, or when tossing and turning at night, when things didn't go my way, when I'd left an 'I-don't-feel-right-here' situation or after ending a toxic relationship. I wondered so many times why my life was the way it was.

At some level we all suffer from low self-esteem – a lack of self-confidence. When the mind goes to that dark place, we start to miss out on opportunities and many of the wonderful things in life because we would rather avoid engaging with anything and anyone.

At the core of these issues is a statement that we start to believe: I am not good enough. We believe that we don't deserve any type of happiness and that we are going to have, at best, a mediocre life. When we think like this, it's a sure sign of low self-esteem.

Imposter Syndrome

The concept of Imposter Syndrome ties in with this idea of not being good enough. It refers to the idea of feeling like a fraud, and is especially prevalent in the workplace. If you find yourself questioning your accomplishments, wondering if you deserve your successes or the good things in your life or feeling like you don't measure up to those around you, then you are more than likely afflicted by this. But you should know that you are not alone.

It is easy to fall into the trap of feeling like an imposter, especially as we are increasingly bombarded with images and ideas of perfection from different media. Even the most successful people have been known to suffer with this syndrome, and it can have quite a debilitating effect on your mood, as well as your desire to continue striving for success.

A lot of the self-doubt that fuels Imposter Syndrome stems from how we feel other people perceive us. We worry that we are being judged or that our abilities aren't as great as they actually are – and that other people know this. This can lead us to believe that we are inadequate and don't deserve to have a great life.

Moving On From Negative Self-talk

This month is all about turning around those feelings of inadequacy by learning how to rebuild your self-esteem once and for all. When you do so, you will walk out of your home and into this great big, wide world holding your head high! Self-esteem is about having confidence in you – no one else but *you*.

I used to have a habit, or really a pattern, whereby I would internalise anything and everything anyone said about me, whether to my face, via email or text. I would think about it all day, and then all week. If it was constructive criticism, I certainly would not take it that way. Instead, I twisted it into something bad, something negative, and drew the conclusion that something was wrong with me. And if someone said something nice about me, I wouldn't believe it! I would think they were just trying to be nice, and that they actually felt the opposite about me. Good or bad, I was internalising it, paranoid about what was said, or what it all meant, creating false beliefs about myself. Basically, in my own head I was making stuff up that wasn't true.

Not surprisingly, my self-esteem started to deteriorate and I began to lose my sense of self. I didn't know who I was any more because I chose to believe the stories in my head.

I think that nearly everyone, to some degree, wants to learn how to truly develop their self-esteem. And that's why this month is all about *rebuilding*.

Self-esteem Vs Ego

People sometimes confuse high self-esteem with having a big ego or being narcissistic. This is especially the case if the person in question is a woman. But, there is a *big* difference. People with healthy self-esteem are secure with who they are – imperfections and all. In fact, they love their imperfections, because they understand that they are what makes them unique.

As you start to rebuild your self-esteem, you will soon realise that no one is perfect. In fact, when you meet a seemingly 'perfect' person, you will soon discover that they are in constant need of approval. I found that once I started to just be me, authentically imperfect me, people began to appreciate me more. Yes, I definitely have flaws, but I have learned to work on them and still love them.

When you become more confident, rebuilding your self-esteem, it will be as if a huge weight has been lifted off your shoulders. You'll start to feel secure, confident and light as a feather! And this can rapidly impact all areas of your life: you will see a difference in how you interact with your colleagues, how you behave in your relationships and also how open you are to dealing with strangers.

Once the weight has been lifted, you can train yourself

to become self-confident over time. Self-confidence will separate you from the crowd; you will have an inner glow that radiates from within you. Self-confidence definitely does not need the approval of others. And that is what this month is all about: retraining the brain and establishing self-confidence for life – because, with practice, you'll become more attractive and fun to be around and your outlook on life will become much more positive. There is a saying that 'confidence is contagious', and it's true! Your self-confidence will infect others, too.

Suppressing Feelings

Naturally our self-esteem is strongly influenced by our feelings. Most of us suppress or hide our feelings that we're somehow not good enough, or we aren't honest about them. By not letting our feelings out, we are, obviously, containing them, but doing so creates massive internal frustration.

It is one thing to vent to a friend or family member (which is totally great), but it is another thing to be heard. And to be heard by you! You need to tell yourself on a daily basis that you *are* good enough and you need to listen to yourself – to *hear* yourself, so that you can rebuild your self-esteem.

Being honest with ourselves about how we truly feel about ourselves is step one. It is a sign of strength, not weakness.

Try telling someone about one of your 'imperfections' – sharing with someone else earns respect, demonstrates vulnerability and shows others that you are human. Once we are honest with ourselves, and say, 'I am not confident in who I am', then we can go deeper.

I have to stress that the process of rebuilding self-esteem is about being honest with yourself and not blaming others. Many, many times in my life, I have blamed others. 'He treated me badly and that's the reason I have low self-esteem', or, 'She puts me down and is so critical of me every time I see her', or, 'My whole life, no one has ever said anything nice about me'. The blame game goes on and on.

This might be something that resonates with you. Maybe you've been treated badly, have had toxic relationships in your life (which I hope you are now going to set boundaries around) and perhaps you actually do think that no one has ever really said something nice about you (I genuinely doubt that, but we will be looking more at that inner critic in Month Eight). Regardless, you need to stop blaming others and work on yourself.

Blame will get you nowhere – in fact, blame just creates more resentments, more frustrations and more self-esteem issues. Once you stop blaming, you can get to know yourself again – because if you have been blaming others, you've been focusing on them and not you. So let's put the people that you have been blaming to one side. Instead, I want you to focus on *you*. I know that there are fabulous things about you because we all have totally unique and amazing strengths.

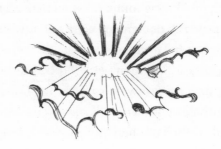

SELF-CARE ACTION: Things I like about me

Write down what you like about yourself, but not what people say they like about you (that's different, although those qualities might also appear on your list):

Flaws as Strengths

Remember, sometimes what you or other people may perceive as a 'flaw' is, in fact, a strength.

Let's say someone said to me, 'You're so opinionated!' That person might have been pointing out what they perceived as a flaw, but when I take a hard look at myself, I like that I have a voice, an opinion. As long as I state my opinion in a loving and kind way, well, that's a trait I should be proud of, not embarrassed about. You see where I'm going with this? I want you to start getting comfortable in your own skin. You don't have to be the person your parents or anyone else wants you to be. Only once you start recognising your own uniqueness, and accepting that there is only one of you here in this world, can you begin to be confident in who you are. You need to embrace the miracle of who you are, starting this month.

Signs of Low Self-esteem

People with low self-esteem often try to hide their imperfections by trying to be 'perfect', which only makes their lives more difficult, stressful and exhausting. They end up keeping secrets and holding back on their true feelings and thoughts – they hide their genuine, authentic selves.

Let's look at the typical signs of low self-esteem. It is one thing to say it, but it is another thing to really dig deep and look at what is happening inside you, feelings and all. On page 85 we'll then look at what you can do to change those feelings.

Accepting Toxic Relationships

Do you have any toxic relationships with people around you? You know, the people who drain your energy – aka energy vampires. Have you ever had a conversation, whether in person or on the phone, and come away feeling as if all of your energy has been zapped; feeling low, not good enough and, well, like your life sucks? Basically, you give and give, while they keep taking and taking. They walk away feeling great, because subconsciously (or otherwise) they know they made you feel less than.

We can't have control over every single relationship that comes into our lives, but we do have control over how much energy we invest in each of them. If we start to spend too much time with these 'energy vampires', then we can become conditioned to think that true, authentic friends don't really exist and this is somehow acceptable or as good as it gets.

When you listen to your gut feeling, you know that you deserve better. You need to trust yourself that you will find the type of relationship you deserve elsewhere – the type of two-way relationship with a friend, co-worker or partner where the energy between you is equal and positive and each of you makes the other feel good. These are the interactions you walk away from feeling confident and happy.

Blaming luck, not talent

The second sign of low self-esteem is thinking that anything good in your life is the result of luck. You find it very hard to come up with a single achievement and, if you do 'say it out loud', you quickly dismiss it, saying something along the lines of, 'Well, I mean, I was just lucky' – as if it wasn't down to your hard work or your drive, or your many talents. Instead, you believe that it was just the universe, for once, looking after you.

Well, ahem ... you're wrong! You totally rocked your achievements on your own, without any interference from so-called luck. Failing to recognise this and be proud of your achievements can seriously affect your self-esteem. It has a knock-on effect on your drive and determination to work towards future goals and dreams, and your passions.

People pleasing

Do you feel you always need to please others and prove yourself – to convince them that you are good enough or smart enough, even though you actually don't believe in your abilities or talents or gifts anyway? Yup, that's another sign of low self-esteem.

Ignoring your dreams

You might have what you think are far-out dreams or aspirations that you wouldn't be caught dead sharing with anyone because you think they are silly, not worthy of anyone's time and maybe others will laugh at you. Dreams are meant for those especially 'gifted' people, which you are definitely not. And even if a dream of yours does constantly pop into your head, and into your heart, you can come up with a million excuses as to why it is silly, stupid and can never be achieved.

But dreams are the things that help you live up to your true potential, your highest self. I'm not talking about those far-fetched ones, like living on a 500-foot, five-storey yacht, travelling the world and never having to work again – those are fantasies. Dreams are the directions in life that you want to follow, what you want to do, aspirations that keep popping back into your head, ideas that you are passionate about. But without self-esteem, it's impossible to realise those dreams.

Difficulty dealing with disappointment

Disappointments are an inevitable part of life, what's important is how you deal with them. Think about a time when you have been disappointed. Maybe you lost your job, had a bad break-up or that new diet didn't work? What happened to your self-esteem at those times? I suspect it went from bad to worse. And those of us with low self-esteem will always find it much harder to get back up. We start to think, 'Well, of course this happened because nothing ever goes right for me'. And, rather than trying to pick ourselves up, we stay down for longer than most, unable to muster up the courage or the strength to try again. We can't understand that whatever it is happened for a reason and that our setbacks inevitably make us stronger.

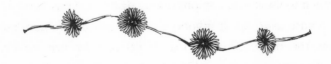

How to Build Your Self-esteem

OK, so let's work on building your self-esteem so that you can start every single day thinking, 'Yup, I *am* good enough. In fact, I'm more than good enough. I'm the only amazing me in this world, and I'm going to live with the self-confidence of being my unique, interesting and incredible self every single day'.

Let go of toxic relationships

For starters, we are going to let go of those toxic relationships we touched on earlier, or at least create healthy boundaries around them. Start by listing those relationships below.

SELF-CARE ACTION:
Identify your toxic relationships

List your toxic relationships/energy vampires here:

When we have connections that make us nervous, anxious or cause us to not feel good about ourselves, we may put way too much effort into them because we are seeking some sort of validation from them, causing us to lose our own power and control. How often do you look to your friends, or those around you, to make you feel good about yourself?

Self-confident people never walk over other people's feelings. Yes, they confidently assert themselves and they have a voice, but their voice and feelings are never heated or overly emotional. Self-confident people are not judgemental or critical, and they accept others and all their flaws, just like they accept themselves, warts and all.

Spend time with positive people

Starting today, spend time with the people who appreciate you. I can tell you first-hand that this is super-essential for your health and happiness and, of course, your self-esteem.

We all deserve to be treated well. And, in my view, if anyone makes you feel 'less than', then that person needs to be kept at arm's length. This is called having 'healthy boundaries' and means that you can have space to be you and do what you want.

You don't have to be there for everyone. It might come as a shock that I'm writing this, and believe in it, but I do; in any relationship, once you feel that you are losing who you are, losing your authentic real self, then you're no longer building your self-worth – you are losing it, fast!

SELF-CARE ACTION: List your true supporters

At the top of the page opposite, list the people in your life who make you feel good about yourself.

Celebrate Your Talents

The following questions can help you to understand your amazing qualities that the world can also see! Answer them as honestly as you can, and try to consider how these things should positively impact your self-esteem:

QUESTIONNAIRE: What's great about you?

- What do you like about you?

- What do you do well?

- What do others say you do well?

- What are the strengths that make you stand out from others?

- What accomplishments come easily to you that maybe aren't easy for others?

You are not being self-absorbed when you say what you like about yourself. When we tell ourselves the things we do well, the things that we like about ourselves and what others like about us too, we are investing in our self-esteem. We are refilling our tank. We are not going to let ourselves run on empty any more.

Visualisation For Self-esteem

Self-esteem means believing in yourself every single day, knowing that you are unique and believing that that's a wonderful thing. Visualisation is a great tool that has massively helped me to rebuild my self-esteem.

When you wake up in the morning, you might think about the day ahead – all that you have to do, all that you want to try to squeeze in, your to-do lists, the people you will be interacting with . . . But now I want you to wake up and think of your day in a different, more confident way.

SELF-CARE ACTION: Visualise a confident you

- Start by visualising yourself walking tall and proud to work, or on the school run or on your errands.

- Visualise yourself speaking with confidence to every-one you meet that day, as you interact with people that make you feel good about yourself.
- Think about how you will feel at the end of the day when you act this way.

Each morning, give yourself permission to be true to who *you* are, not the person others think you should be. Every morning, make a decision to leave your home totally 100 per cent confident in who you are.

As you start to become more confident, you won't need others to validate that confidence for you. Knowing who you are is what this journey is all about. You don't ever have to apologise for having healthy self-esteem. And trust me, your healthy and newly rebuilt self-esteem will help you to attract other positive people and wonderful opportunities.

Failure and Success

If you ever find yourself wondering how a certain individual is so successful, then I can tell you that it's usually down to a lot of hard work, but also a strong sense of self. They keep doing, keep believing and, therefore, keep achieving. They set the bar high and expect to win.

I also believe that failure is winning. Failure teaches you. It puts you on a different path. So ask yourself – where do you set your daily bar? Is it so low so that you won't have any disappointments?

Do any of the following statements sound familiar?

'I already tried that and failed, so I won't ever try again.'

'I lost last time, so I'm sure I'll lose this time.'

'I haven't achieved anything yet, so I'm sure I never will.'

The more you put yourself down, the more you will be sucked into a downward spiral of always 'losing'. But the more you believe in who you are as a unique person, the more your self-confidence will evolve and the more you will win. Self-confident people are not afraid of making mistakes. They see them as an opportunity to learn, and as valuable lessons that can empower them; in fact, they understand that we can actually learn more from our mistakes and failures than from our successes. This is how they get to where they want to be – because mistakes can and will get you to the success you are trying to achieve, but only if you look at them as lessons. And that's why self-confident people are never afraid to keep moving forwards and try again.

Positive Affirmations

Here's a test: think back to as many holidays as you can remember. Now, which do you remember the most? I bet it's the ones where something went wrong. Our brains are wired to remember negative thoughts, emotions, people and situations much more than positive ones. But we can retrain them to think positively about ourselves and our lives. Notice those negative thoughts that bring your self-esteem down, take a breath and stop. Notice as soon as someone else says something that is not helping you feel good about yourself, and replace it with something positive.

SELF-CARE ACTION:
Replace negative thoughts with positive affirmations

I can't live without positive affirmations. Here are some that I suggest you start saying daily. You can either choose to do so first thing in the morning, in order to start your day with a burst of positivity, or you can use them when you notice that negative thoughts are beginning to infiltrate. Say them to yourself a minimum of three times, especially when a negative thought or feeling comes into your mind.

- I am an intelligent person who is competent and confident.

- I believe in my potential and in myself.
- I recognise and admire my own good qualities.
- I always try to see the best in other people.
- Everybody I spend my time with is a positive influence on my life and my character.
- Negative thoughts and feelings about myself have no purpose and I release them.
- I love who I am and I am excited for who I will become.
- I am constantly evolving and growing as a person.
- My opinions are consistent with what I believe in.
- My behaviour is in harmony with who I am and who I want to be.

Be sure to choose the affirmations that resonate the most with you. They might – and probably will – change on a weekly or even a daily basis. You could also perhaps use these affirmations as a starting point to create some more of your own.

Meditation for Self-esteem

Meditation can play a huge role in boosting your self-esteem. My suggestion is to use the following meditation every single day throughout this month. By the end of the month your self-esteem will be radiating outwards for everyone to see and feel!

SELF-CARE ACTION: A simple daily meditation

- Lie down on your sofa or your bed with your knees bent and the soles of your feet flat on the floor.
- Knock your knees in towards each other so that they are lightly touching. This position should feel good on your lower back.
- Close your eyes, as this immediately helps to calm the central nervous system, getting you out of fight/ flight/freeze mode (see page 37), all of which massively affects our self-esteem.
- Scan your body and feel where you might be holding tension: begin with your feet, move up to the ankles, lower legs, knees, upper legs, hips, abdomen, sides of the waist, chest, lower back, middle back, upper back, shoulders, throat, jaw, cheeks, eye sockets, eyebrows, forehead, back of the head and the top of the head ...
- *... and then just let it go.*
- Bring your focus to your breath, and as you inhale, breathe in self-confidence, and as you exhale, breathe out self-doubt.
- Do twelve rounds of breathing in this way.

Inhale self-confidence, exhale self-doubt. Inhale self-confidence, exhale self-doubt. Do twelve full breaths as you silently repeat those words.

More Useful Tips

Visualisation, positive affirmations and meditation are great ways to help rebuild your self-esteem. I urge you to do these three things every single day throughout this month.

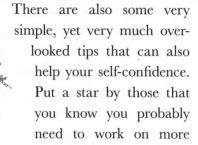

There are also some very simple, yet very much overlooked tips that can also help your self-confidence. Put a star by those that you know you probably need to work on more than others.

- Start looking others in the eye when having conversations.
- Observe other people; you will start to see that everyone is unique – including you.
- Start saying 'no' to people or situations that do not help your self-esteem.
- Walk with confidence, knowing that you are one of a kind.
- Accept compliments (don't volley them back). Smile and say 'thank you'.
- Stop putting yourself down. If your past wasn't positive, then decide today what your future will be by saying positive things about yourself.

- Don't try to be someone else or wish you were. Comparison robs you of your self-esteem.
- Make decisions throughout your day that make you feel good about yourself.
- Make daily deposits in your self-esteem bank and stop withdrawing.
- Own your confidence.
- Stop your doubts from becoming debilitating. Your contribution to this world is unique.
- Smile – and make it confident and genuine.
- Focus on what you want in life. If you focus on what might not work, it won't. Keep a positive outlook on what you want out of your future.
- Be persistent.
- Change the way you treat yourself through positive self-talk and your actions.

Ultimately, only you can help yourself on the path to strong self-esteem. I have given you the tools this month that have helped me. If you use them and commit to a practice every single day, your self-esteem will increase, day by day. You will soon notice that you have self-confidence in every situation, no matter what you're faced with.

Month Five

Alleviating Anxiety

Be gentle with yourself.
You're doing the best you can.

ANONYMOUS

Statistics show that women are twice as likely as men to suffer from anxiety, and it has been estimated that it's a problem affecting up to 16 per cent of the population at any one time. Generalised Anxiety Disorder (GAD), where the sufferer is in a constant state of high anxiety, is one of the most common types of anxiety, and up to 5 per cent of the population are struggling with it. However, GAD accounts for approximately 30 per cent of mental-health related visits to the doctor.

The number of people who connect their anxiety to financial concerns could be as high as 67 per cent, according to one study. And more than 20 per cent of people have abused alcohol in order to cope with feelings of anxiety. The long-term implications of doing this can be extremely worrying for both mental and physical health, and can be detrimental to many other areas of a person's life. Worryingly, many people are more likely to Google their symptoms when they are suffering from a mental-health problem, such as anxiety, rather than speak to their GP about it. This can not only lead to misinformation but is also very unlikely to help with any underlying issues.

Anxiety can vary in severity from person to person. It can be anything from a mild, niggling feeling to a full-blown emotionally crippling issue. Most of us have experienced some level of anxiety – big or small – at some point in our lives, so we know that it certainly isn't fun at all.

I can't put this strongly enough: if you are affected by anxiety on a daily basis and feel that it is affecting your ability to cope with life, please visit your GP.

Coping With Anxiety

The good news is that there are natural – aka non-prescription – ways to deal with anxiety. And that's what this month is all about: utilising natural tools that work – and work well – to help lessen, and perhaps even eliminate, feelings of anxiety.

If you struggle with anxiety, finding ways to soften it will help you to continue on the path of confidence in your own self-worth that you set out on last month. It will also help you to navigate your way through difficult decisions in all areas of your life.

I have suffered with anxiety in the past, and whenever it crept up on me, I felt as though I couldn't breathe. I even felt nauseous. And I was also afraid. I didn't know what was happening to my body: my heart was beating fast, I was sweating and I felt dizzy and confused. That was a case of intense anxiety. I have also had bouts of mild anxiety, whereby I felt impatient and just needed to leave the situation that I was in or the person I was with. I wanted to get home as quickly as possible and curl up under my duvet, shutting everything and everyone out.

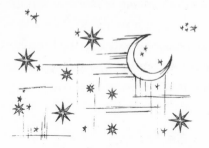

I didn't like these feelings at all, so I did a lot of research and 'road tested' simple but effective ways to help me stop, or at least lessen, them when they surfaced. I managed to work small moments of anxiety-specific self-care into my everyday life, and what a difference these small moments made: I stopped experiencing anxiety at any level.

Now, I can cope – and cope well – when I feel any sort

of anxiety trying to rear its head. I know what to do. My self-care tips are now second nature to me. And the same can be true for you. You just need to make a habit of it. In this chapter I'll share all of the actions that I am referring to when I speak of these life-changing small moments of self-care that reduce anxiety.

Understanding Your Anxiety

Whether you have had high or low levels of anxiety, it is still anxiety, although it is different for all of us. Some of us have lived with it for years, maybe since childhood, whereas others have only experienced it in adulthood.

As I said, I suffered from both high- and low-level anxiety, and I learned that it stemmed from a root 'problem'. If that root can be not only discovered but also dug up and analysed, it can be controlled, softened and even healed. This is because usually anxiety is trying to teach us something that we need to learn or overcome.

QUESTIONNAIRE: What is your anxiety trying to tell you?

When you experience some level of anxiety, ask yourself the following:

- What triggered it?

- Who triggered it?

- What are you feeling – physically, mentally and emotionally?

Anxiety is just a response to our fears, to a perceived threat which causes our fight/flight/freeze stress response to kick in (see page 37).

Now, think back to a time where you felt your anxiety bubbling to the surface and you simply wanted to escape, to get away from wherever you were and whoever you were with. Describe it here:

Listening to what your anxiety is trying to tell you is the best way to begin addressing it. This can guide you to discovering the underlying issue that your mind is trying to make you aware of. The next step is to either avoid it or listen to this guidance and go towards it.

Addressing Lifestyle Triggers

Anxiety is often triggered by our lifestyle. We can help to decrease our levels of anxiety by looking more closely at how we live, what we eat, how we exercise and how we take care of ourselves.

Diet

When I started to cut things out of my diet and also to add things in, I noticed a shift right away in my anxious tendencies.

So what did I cut out?

Caffeine, sugar and alcohol

These three things can actually cause feelings of anxiety. Caffeine is a stimulant that can inhibit the chemicals in the brain that induce sleep, as well as increasing adrenaline production. It can take the body as long as six hours to eliminate caffeine from the body, which is not good news for your sleep cycle if you have consumed it in the late afternoon or evening.

Sugar and alcohol can have the same effects, so watch your sugar, caffeine and alcohol intake and perhaps eliminate them altogether.

If you do sometimes consume one or more of these three things, remind yourself of the effect they can have on you, but don't beat yourself up about it. The point here is to be honest with yourself. If that anxiety does rear its head the next day, you will know that it's most likely caused by one of these three culprits. For example, the lack of sleep you experience might have been brought on by the double espresso you had after dinner. That is your underlying issue. That is your anxiety talking. And you need to start listening.

Tips to Recharge: Foods to Combat Anxiety

I also mentioned adding foods into your diet to help combat anxiety. When you feel that anxiety begin to creep up, here are some great foods to have close at hand!

- **Herbal tea** Make a cup of tea as soon as you feel that anxiousness bubbling at the surface. But not just any cup of tea. There are certain herbs that can help promote sensations of calm and reduce anxiety levels. I once visited a herbal doctor in London, and he explained that nervines are herbs that can be used to help with mild anxiety, and of course, stress. Look for nervine tea that contains one or a mixture of the following: lavender, lemon balm, passion flower, chamomile, oat straw and verbena. These nervines can help nourish a depleted and weakened nervous system. And the good news is that there are lots of amazing tea varieties now available that include many of the herbs listed above.
- **Dark leafy greens** You've got your calming drink sorted, but you should also include anxiety-reducing foods in your diet. The foods we are looking at to help with anxiety are rich in magnesium – a strong, calming mineral. And many of us are deficient in magnesium, so there's another good reason to get more of these foods in. Dark leafy greens, like spin-ach, kale and Swiss chard are full of magnesium.

Make it a habit over this next month to include these in your diet every single day – in a salad at lunch or as a side for dinner.

- **Nuts and seeds** Keep some nuts and seeds at your desk or in your handbag. You can hit your daily quota of magnesium by eating just half a cup of pumpkin seeds! And, of course, you can also include cashews, flaxseeds, pecans, sunflower seeds, almonds and Brazil nuts – all of these are loaded with magnesium too. Try making a trail mix of all of these to keep your energy levels up and your anxiety low.

- **Legumes** Soybeans, black beans, chickpeas, lentils and kidney beans are all rich in magnesium. As with nuts and seeds and dark green leafy veg, make it a habit this month to get some legumes into your diet every single day too. Hummus, dhal, black-bean burgers or chilli are some easy suggestions.

- **Avocados and other fruits** My favourite of favourites – avocado! I don't care that it is the most over-photographed food on social media; it is still my favourite because it is loaded with vitamins and is undeniably one of the most nutritious foods around. One avocado gives you 15 per cent of the recommended daily amount of magnesium. Perfect! Moving on, while bananas are renowned for their potassium, they also have a good amount of magnesium and can easily be popped into your bag for an on-the-go snack. Other fruits with good levels of magnesium are grapefruit, figs and blackberries.

- **Dark chocolate** And last, but certainly not least, dark chocolate! Yes, you can have dark chocolate (70 per cent cocoa or higher) to boost your magnesium intake, which, in turn, counteracts anxiety. So how about combining a few squares of dark chocolate with some blackberries for an anxiety-busting hit?

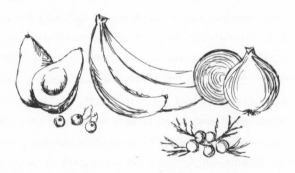

If you look at what to eat to counter anxiety, it's actually pretty simple, not to mention delicious. Get some sort of salad in daily, along with a handful of nuts and seeds, add some beans to your salad or some hummus for a snack, pop an avocado in your salad too or enjoy it on toast in the morning. Have that banana for your snack, or chuck one in a smoothie and it's not too hard to have some dark chocolate on hand either! Pretty simple. You just need to make it happen every day this month, so that it becomes a healthy habit for life.

At the back of the book you'll find a blank 7-day food diary, where you can record what you eat – to ensure you are including plenty of this good stuff (see page 253–5).

Yoga

Yoga is quite possibly my favourite thing in the world, bar my family! You see, I believe yoga 'saved' me – from heading into a deep, dark depression, from being anxious all the time and from super-charged stress levels during those hard years. It's what got me back to the point of loving who I was and who I am. And yoga can do the same for you.

The hardest thing about yoga is actually turning up on your mat. Yes, it's true. And it is not just about being flexible – yoga is *so* much more than just a collection of poses.

Studies have shown that those of us with anxiety might have diminished activity in the brain's GABA systems. Gamma-amino butryric acid (GABA) is an amino acid that acts as the main neurotransmitter in the brain. It essentially helps to soothe our nerves, bringing us back to a calmer state, so that we can function better. And guess what? Yoga increases GABA levels in the brain. One study found that people who practised yoga for an hour experienced a 27 per cent increase in GABA levels compared to zero increase within a control group who read for an hour. And all this without some pill with potentially scary side effects.

Unlike some prescribed medications, practising yoga

regularly doesn't numb your emotions – it helps you to *feel* them. And even better news? There are no negative side effects, besides the very slight possibility of mildly injuring yourself if you enter or hold a pose incorrectly. And that's very rare.

Yoga also helps to decrease your heart rate, keep breathing at a normal pace and lowers blood pressure. Why? Because when you do yoga, you perform other wonderful exercises like controlled breathing, mindfulness and yes, meditation. Savasana – the pose you lie in at the end of a class – is a form of meditation.

So what are you waiting for? Just put on some loose, comfortable clothes, breathe and start moving your body! If you can't make it to a yoga class there are some great, free classes online, you just need to do a quick search. Otherwise, I find that just five poses (Child's Pose, Bound-angle Pose, Tree Pose, Legs-up-the-wall Pose and Camel Pose) – with the inclusion of breathing for five breaths in each one, staring off into space (meditation) and watching yourself breathe for those five breaths (mindfulness) – really help to alleviate anxiety. And no, they are not difficult either. As I said, yoga is so much more than just poses.

All of these poses are very good hip openers – and hip openers are a fantastic way to release any deep-seated emotions and feelings that just might be triggering your anxiety. Will yoga completely eliminate anxiety from your life for ever? Probably not. But neither will any pill. We are all human, after all, and life throws us many curveballs.

What regular practice can do is to help us cope better when life presents us with those inevitable challenges.

SELF-CARE ACTION: Five fantastic yoga poses

Child's Pose
- Begin on your hands and knees on your mat, with your knees hip-width apart and your big toes touching.
- Next, sit up straight and, as you sit back on to your heels, feel your spine lengthen.
- Exhale and bend forwards so that your torso is between your thighs.
- Extend your arms straight in front of you to rest with your palms flat on the floor.
- Breathe for five breaths or more.

Bound-angle Pose
- Begin in a seated position, feet flat on the floor, knees bent. Now bend your knees out to the side as you bring the soles of your feet together.
- Interlace your fingers around your toes and breathe out as you draw your hips down and stretch your head up towards the sky.
- Your shoulders should be down and back, and your chest should be pressed forwards.
- Keep your hips open by continuing to draw your knees down into the floor.

- Exhale and look upwards.
- Breathe for five full breaths.

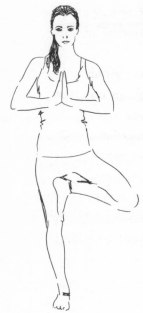

Tree Pose
- Begin by standing before bending the right knee and moving all of your body weight onto your left leg.
- Position your right knee to face away from you to the right, as you rest your heel against your left leg.
- Focus your gaze on a point in front of you as you slide your right foot up your left leg, until you reach a comfortable position where you can maintain your balance.
- Bring your palms together in prayer position in front of your body.
- Breathe for five full breaths.

Legs-up-the-wall Pose
- Start this pose by lying flat on the floor with the left side of your body against the wall.
- Gently turn your body to the left and swing your legs up flat against the wall.
- Shuffle your weight from side to side to bring your buttocks as close to the wall as possible.
- Close your eyes and breathe for five full breaths.

Camel Pose

- Begin by resting on your knees hip-width apart on your mat.
- The palms of your hands should be resting at the base of your spine with your fingers pointing towards the floor.
- Breathe in as you draw your knees over your hips and lengthen your spine upwards through the crown of your head.
- Squeeze your buttocks and thighs together as you bend your body backwards and slowly reach down to grab your heels.
- Drop your head back as far as is comfortably possible.
- Keep your hips forwards and over your knees and lift your chest.
- Breathe for five full breaths.

Mindfulness

Mindfulness is an effective way to cope with and lower the impact of anxiety. It helps us to reconnect the body and mind, and to better understand the sensations and feelings that we experience. It brings us back into the present moment and discourages unhelpful, unnecessary negativity.

At a basic level, becoming mindful can be achieved simply by taking a moment to become aware of your thoughts, noticing how your body feels and stopping to observe what is going on around you. This is useful for tackling anxiety because the very act of doing this will mean that you are less, if at all, able to focus on your anxiety. And the less power and attention you give to the anxious feelings, the more they will reduce, allowing you to rebalance your mind in that moment. And the more we can repeat that awareness of reality, moment by moment, the less 'room' we have in our minds for worry and anxiety about what has gone before or what the future holds for us.

The importance of gratitude

One practice that really helps me to stay present and grounded is gratitude. When I first read about a gratitude practice, I was sceptical to the point of being anti-gratitude! I thought it was going to be one of the 'next big' wellness tips that fades away and loses steam as quickly as it arrives. But I was wrong. Having read numerous articles and books about the benefits of practising gratitude – one of them being to reduce anxiety levels, I just had to try it out for myself to see a) if it really worked and b) what the hype was all about. And now? I am here to attest to the fact that a) it does *really* work and b) I can see and feel what all the hype was about!

My initial reason for adopting a gratitude practice was because of my tendency towards anxiety, but I soon realised that it has so many more benefits. Filling my life with gratitude by frequently making the conscious decision to express thanks for the things I appreciate has meant I've built better and stronger relationships with those I love, and I feel less stressed and more confident. Practising gratitude has also helped to release many of my fears, which were created by me and only existed in my head.

Getting started with mindfulness gratitude
So how and what do you start with?

I have done a lot of written gratitude practices, whereby you write letters to those in your life who have meant and done something positive to you or for you. You can send the letter or choose not to; the point is simply to write it. It works! And it's truly satisfying – the oxytocin (love hormone) kicks in, and you feel *great* afterwards.

Another practice that I still do to this day is to write or even mentally say three things that I am grateful for every night before bed. Again, I feel happy after I do this – the oxytocin gets going and I sleep well. But this month, we are going to go a bit deeper with our habit-forming gratitude practice and make a daily healthy habit that really sticks.

Breathing, meditation and mindfulness
This month you are going to learn how to incorporate these key well-being practices into one exercise for alleviating anxiety. While the exercise combines all three practices, it doesn't require you to be in any particular pose or position. This triple combo is designed to put your parasympathetic nervous system (the calm one, see page

50) in the driving seat and not your sympathetic nervous system (the crazy one). You can do it anywhere, anytime – even during a heated discussion!

SELF-CARE ACTION: Calming triple combo

- Start by immediately zooming in on your breath. You can still talk and carry on a conversation as you focus on your breathing.
- After just a few breaths, start to count your inhale. It might be just two to three seconds long. That's OK. I just want you to count your inhale.
- Next, count your exhale while still counting your inhale. So, you might be two to three seconds on the inhale and two to three seconds on the exhale. Just keep counting both the inhale and the exhale for the next few breaths.
- Now, I want you to lengthen the inhale by one second and lengthen the exhale by two seconds, so that your exhale becomes a little bit longer than your inhale. Keep counting.
- Do this for three more breaths.
- Lastly, we are going to do that one more time. Again, lengthen your inhale by one second and your exhale by two seconds. So now your exhale should be two seconds longer than your inhale.
- Again, do this for three more breaths.

Continue if it feels good. You will get to the point where you do not need to count your breath any more because you now know what it feels like. Once you feel your breath and don't need to count any more, you can start to add words to your inhale and exhale. Some good examples are:

- Inhale 'I am' and exhale 'totally calm'.
- Inhale 'I am' and exhale 'practising self-care'.
- Inhale 'Self-care' and exhale 'is my priority'.

Write these down and keep them in your back pocket so that they are at your fingertips when you need them. Try doing this breathing exercise at least once a day throughout this month to make it a healthy habit that you can call on at literally a moment's notice.

And, just for good measure, here are some other examples that are very effective:

- Inhale: 'Let'; exhale: 'go'
- Inhale: 'I take'; exhale: 'care of me'
- Inhale: 'My body'; exhale: 'is relaxing'
- Inhale: 'I am practising'; exhale: 'taking care of me'
- Inhale: 'I am'; exhale: 'totally calm'
- Inhale: 'I am'; exhale: 'practising self-care'
- Inhale: 'Self-care'; exhale: 'is my priority'
- Inhale: 'I release'; exhale: 'all worry'

SELF-CARE ACTION: Be thankful for your day

Just before bed (because we all have to end up in bed every night, so there should be no excuse not to do this), ask yourself how you are feeling. There is no right or wrong answer. You could be feeling awful or you could be feeling satisfied. You are just acknowledging how you are feeling.

- How are you feeling right now?
- Next, focus on the things in your life right now that make you happy. (Some nights you may only come up with one thing; yes, I am sure there are plenty more, but we all have those kind of nights!) Whatever you come up with – whether it's one thing or a multitude of things – just say thank you after each one.
- What made you happy today? What makes you happy now?
- Now, take a look at what you struggled with in your day. Perhaps you lost your temper, had mood swings, didn't eat well – trust me, we all have these moments. The point is to stop shoving these struggles under a rug and hiding them. We need to say thank you to them as well! Perhaps they have taught you a lesson or you have found a silver lining through them. Perhaps the silver lining has not revealed itself to you just yet (it will, it just takes time and patience), but be sure to say thank you to what you struggled with in your day.

- Lastly, you need to end with five breaths. On the inhale, say, 'Thank you' to everything you just listed in your head or on paper, and on the exhale say, 'For it all'.

Try not to abandon this gratitude practice when anxiety kicks in – because no matter what your day is like, there is *always* something to be grateful for, even if it is just the roof over your head or the food you have to eat. If you learn to take the time to be grateful after each and every day, no matter what it entailed, and make that a habit, you might soon find that it transforms your life.

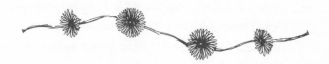

Sally's Story

Sally, a student of mine, challenged herself to remove some-thing negative from her life to make more space to receive the positive. Here's what happened:

'I chose to eliminate negative thoughts by maintaining a daily gratitude journal. Brene Brown, author of *Rising Strong*, said that she didn't like or agree with the sweeping phrase, "attitude of gratitude", as gratitude is not so much an attitude that we can just switch on, but a daily practice – a discipline. So my discipline has turned into writing out as many things that I am grateful for as I can come up with at the end of each and every day. (It is important to include the "why" as well, to avoid just listing without emotion.) I make it my mission to write as I get into bed every night, regardless of time, jet lag, drunkenness, my fiancé wanting to get it on, you name it!

'At one point, a dear friend who was going through a difficult time asked me, in all sincerity, if I really could come up with something to be grateful for every single day. It broke my heart. The truth is, when we are going through tough times, we lose sight of the countless things we have to be grateful for. My list has included things as simple as being able to live in a vibrant city like London, a sunny day (it *is* London, after all), a healthy meal, taking a yoga class, the kindness of strangers (seeing people give up their seat on the Underground always restores my faith in humanity) and so on.

'I started the practice of "an attitude to gratitude" by saying thank you in my head three times after things I was truly grateful for; two most common instances are after *namaste* in a yoga class and every single time I land safely at a new destination.

'Gratitude will transform your life into a happier, more positive one, but it is a daily practice. *You will soon find that the secret to having it all is realising you already do.*'

SELF-CARE ACTION:
Prompt yourself to be grateful

Write these gratitude reminders down where you will
see them every day this month – you could stick them
to your fridge or write them in your journal. Just make
sure you have them close by, so that they become hard-
wired and you create an ongoing gratitude practice for
the rest of your life.

- Both the act of gratitude and the act of worry are
  optional. Choosing to express gratitude means you
  have less time to worry.
- Expressing gratitude allows you to recognise and
  acknowledge the positivity in your life.
- Every day is a fresh opportunity to discover exciting
  aspects of your life to express gratitude for.
- Worrying about something will not change the out-
  come of the problem; it simply prevents you from
  experiencing happiness in these moments.

Anxiety is a part of living and what I like to call our
'life experiences'. Without these, the ones that make
you really *feel*, you will never grow to your true potential, or find the true, authentic and wonderful you.
However, being able to control your anxiety – through
yoga, healthy eating, meditation and mindfulness – can

change your entire life. I have experienced such a huge shift in my own life by incorporating these simple moments of self-care and I have now reached a place where I am in control of my anxiety, rather than *it* controlling *me*.

Month Six

Finding, Believing In and Building Your Passions

Don't ask what the world needs.
Ask what makes you come alive, and go
do it. Because what the world needs is
people who have come alive.

HOWARD THURMAN

Few people are born knowing what they want to do with their lives, and we should all regularly remind ourselves of this, especially when we are feeling lost or we're experiencing a lack of direction or enthusiasm for life.

A lot of us confuse hobbies and passions. It is true to say that hobbies can and will bring us happiness. They keep us sane, but they're the things we fit in around other stuff. A passion, on the other hand, is something we can't stop thinking about; it's something we feel we absolutely need to do and we have to do whatever we can to make it happen.

A passion could be the urge to invent something, to build a business, to discover something new. It could be connected to your own personal growth or to helping others. It could be education-related, such as gaining a qualification in something that has always excited you, or employment-related, such as obtaining your dream job. It could be all of these things or none of them – and that's the point: it is totally unique to you.

It is true that the journey to discovering your passions can be a long one, with many distractions, hurdles, hardships and diversions along the way, but it is worth it to find them!

Time To Get Unstuck

This month is all about how to get 'unstuck' and find your calling – because, trust me, we *all* have a passion, even if right now you don't think you do. In time, yours will reveal itself to you.

Discovering your passion and embracing it as a serious part of your life is a great way to boost your personal well-being. This is because the new sense of satisfaction and fulfilment you will find in life will guide and enhance your happiness.

In the meantime, you can take some steps to help uncover your passions, little by little. What you are doing today, the path that you are on today and what you are learning from that current path – all of this is a part of the bigger picture. It's a part of discovering your passions, all of which will lead you to your purpose here on earth. Because yes, we do *all* have a purpose. And it is never, *ever* too late for any of us to find, believe in and live our passions.

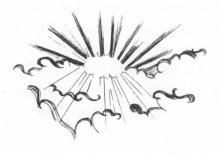

The burning question is, 'How do I find my passion in life?' I did not know what passion was until I started to ask questions. I thought that surely there must be more to life than just going through the motions: wake up, get the kids ready for school, get ready for work, work out, run errands, go to work, have lunch, pick up kids from school, come home from work, make supper, watch TV, go to bed ... I was living for everyone else. I wasn't living for me and I started to become resentful. Sound vaguely familiar?

However, my resentment didn't lie with everyone else, but with me. I started to resent myself because I wasn't doing anything that was important to me. Whatever it was that I cared about was always on the back burner because a) I thought I didn't have time, b) I thought everyone would think it was stupid and c) I thought that everyone else's needs and wants should definitely come before my own.

My passion was there, but so well hidden, so covered by other 'important' things and responsibilities, that it didn't have a chance to 'breathe'. And the same could be true for yours. If it could breathe, if you were to allow it to come up for air, then you would see that there is energy, amazingly strong energy, in your passion – it just needs to be set free.

So, rather than asking ourselves the difficult questions – you know, the 'Why me?' ones – we need to start asking ourselves bigger, better and more empowering questions. These are the questions that really helped me to find my passions. Oh, and remember, you can absolutely have more than one passion.

QUESTIONNAIRE: What do you feel passionate about?

Your passions might have been lost in the pit of your stomach, the depths of your mind or under a bunch of 'other' things that you do for everyone else. But this month is all about uncovering, dusting off and finally making your love of something (aka your passion) a priority.

Let's start with some questions:

- What did I love to do when I was younger?

- When do I feel the happiest?

- What do I do in my life that brings a massive smile to my face?

- What do I do in my life that makes me forget about anything and everything?

- What, in other people, do I love and crave for myself?

- Who inspires me?

- What do I want to be known for?

- When I dream about my life, what am I dreaming I am doing or being?

- When I wake up every morning, how do I want to feel?

- What do I do that comes easily to me?

- What do I do that gives me peace and happiness?

- What idea or goal or dream keeps coming back to me?

- If I could do anything in the world without worrying about anyone or anything else at all, what would it be?

- What do I do that makes me feel me – my most authentic and real me?

- What are the characteristic traits that I value the most about myself?

- What books or subject matter do I always gravitate towards?

- If money was no object, what would I spend the next five or more years creating and doing?

I am certain that when you start answering these questions, more will pop into your head. Write them down and answer those, too. You will find that once you start to truly focus on what it is that you love to do, you can write a thesis about it because you are so passionate about *that* thing!

Positive Change To Inspire Your Passions

Your passion starts out as a tiny seed and may not grow much because it hasn't been watered or loved and nurtured enough – if at all. But once you start taking care of your passion, it will start to grow. And once that happens, there will be no stopping you!

SELF-CARE ACTION: Nurture that creative seed

Each day this month you are going to do something out of the ordinary to help bring your passion to the surface. The point here is to start shifting your mindset by thinking out of the box and, little by little, you will nurture that creative seed.

Here are some suggestions:

- Walk to work.
- Make a juice.
- Wear a pair of shoes from last year.
- Shop at a new supermarket.
- Say hello to a stranger on the street.
- Head to a restaurant in a different part of town.
- Try a new superfood.

Write down your own 'out-of-the-ordinary' suggestions here:

SELF-CARE ACTION:
List your potential passions

Each day this month (if you can), write down one thing per day that you feel could become a real passion – anything from visiting places you have never been before to meeting people you have always wanted to meet, achieving things that you have always wanted to do. The sky's the limit!

Document your passion(s) here:

Do I do this? Absolutely! I have written down many, many times that I would like to meet Oprah Winfrey. I grew up watching her before she became a household name. And now look at her! So, yes, I dream of meeting her, not least because of her wise words: 'Passion is energy. Feel the power that comes from focusing on what excites you.' I also dream of visiting the Galápagos Islands so that Nestor, my youngest, can live his fantasy of being in the natural world! I dream about running a marathon and climbing Mount Kilamanjaro. I dream about working in the Peace Corps. I dream about having my own yoga studio. And I dream about sailing around the world with my husband once our kids are grown.

Will I do all of these things? Maybe. Maybe not. But that's not the point. Within each of my dreams, I then find something that I am passionate about. In doing so I create a tangible goal that I can think about working towards. That is what I want you to do as well.

QUESTIONNAIRE: How can you move forwards?

Once you have a list of your potential passions, contemplate these questions.

- What is it about these things that makes you want to do them?

- Is there a way that you can shape your career around them?

- Can you dedicate some of your spare time to learning more about one of your passions?

Passion Equals Effort

You've probably clocked that some of the passions I mentioned are huge and seemingly impossible. But let me explain why this makes some sort of sense. The word 'passion' actually comes from the Latin word *pati*, meaning 'suffering'. When I first learned that I thought it made no sense, but the more I thought about it, the more I realised it does. Here's why: your passion is something for which you are willing to 'suffer', to go through ups and downs, to learn from difficulties and hardships. Because that's what helps you to realise your passion. And it's an amazing and huge step towards becoming fulfilled.

So you have to ask yourself what you are willing to do to make your passions a reality. Are you willing to put in the time, to pull the all-nighters, if necessary, to work for days straight without a break?

When you write your passions down every day this month I hope you get a real sense of where you want your life to go. When I look at mine, they include self-care (doing something for me), and helping others with their own self-care. What is your gut urging you to do? This month I want you to think about this – dream about it – every single day. Don't stop dreaming!

How Passions Improve Your Well-being

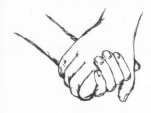 Doing what you love has huge bene-
fits, one of which is that it makes you
feel great. But there is more, oh so much
more, in terms of the health benefits we
experience when we find and pursue
our passions.

Reduced stress levels

As we discussed in Month Two, stress hormones are constantly being released into our bodies (although hopefully,
by now, you have created some great habits to ensure your
cortisol switch is less reactive). However, following your
passions is a great way to switch off stress. Whether their
passion is a blog, a YouTube channel, a charity, healthy
eating, fitness, yoga, cycling, art, jewellery making, fashion
design, a career change or a promotion, most people start
to notice an increase in energy as well as a calm within the
parasympathetic nervous system (see page 50) when they're
immersed in what they love. If we can get into that state
we can stay in that calm rest and digest mode which, of
course, assists in our overall well-being. Have you noticed
that when you are fully immersed in something you are
passionate about, you don't eat as much, or any 'bad'
foods? This is because when you are on a 'high', building
your passions, you are far less stressed. And when you
are less stressed, you don't crave those 'emotional-eating'

foods, such as that tub of ice cream, piece of cake or entire bag of crisps. The excitement around your passions releases those feel-good chemicals (such as dopamine), and when this happens you don't need to use junk food to get that fix any more. Your passion, in effect, becomes your very own tub of ice cream!

Improved mood

That leads me to the next benefit to be considered when you are working towards your passions, and that is that you will be in a much better mood. When you work on what you love, when you do what you love, your body releases endorphins. Your passions generate endorphins, just like other forms of self-care, such as running, yoga, meditation and breathing.

Satisfaction and fulfilment

Think back to your digital detox in Month Three. Finding your passion can help you to keep up with that detox because you will not be bored. You'll have something to do that you love, so you won't need to check what everyone else is doing on Facebook, Twitter and Instagram a hundred times a day. And even if you haven't found your passion yet, remember that this month is all about believing that you have one. Because when you find that something that you love – your passion – it will make you feel more fulfilled, more alive and you will live life to the full.

Mary's Story

Mary, one of my yoga students, wanted so badly to believe she had a passion, to find out what it was and to then start building it. Here's her story:

'Some say that I am chasing the impossible. And frankly, I sometimes feel they might be right. But then, at the most unexpected times, I feel this fire within me, this burning desire to be and do something greater than my life. The only problem is I don't know what that "thing" is. So three years ago I started on a journey to identify my passions and to discover what my life purpose is. I attended workshops, I read books, articles, magazines and I took the personality and career tests.

'Most recently I took a four-day intensive course to help me really feel and find my true passion. I thought, Perfect! The course will just confirm that I should further pursue my hobbies (photography and yoga) and then I'll get the official go-ahead to finally walk away from my corporate job. But oh, wow! That was not the answer. Surprised? Yes, me too. Turns out, photography and yoga were my hobbies, but my passion was to start a company that offers team-building events.

'It's been five months since that course, and I'm still working on the journey. They say that the journey is much more fun than the destination, and I think they're right! I'm getting closer to the answer, and for the first time in my life I'm letting it unfold how it's meant to. I'm trusting the process and I am confident that once I get there, I'll be able to connect the dots. Maybe I'll get there next year, or maybe it will be in ten years. One thing's for sure, I'll learn and grow every step of the way.'

Making the effort to explore your passions, as Mary did, is something that I bet many of you reading this now have never found the time to do. Well, now is your time – this month, right here, right now is where you will begin. Find, believe in and build your passions!

Vision Boarding

A vision board is a collage of cut-out images, sentences and words that reflect the things you want in your life and the person you want to become. Vision boarding is a great way to switch off from everything else and just focus on you, the things you love to do and stoke that fire within you.

Some good examples and things that I have used in the past are inspirational quotes or words, pictures of friends and family members (these do not have to be real pictures of these people – the cut-outs can simply represent them), places you would like to visit, things you would like to have, some of your favourite things in the world, your goals, your dreams, whatever you are grateful for, the things that make you smile, the things you love to do and basically anything that represents you.

I recently made a vision board that represented one particular passion of mine – something I truly wanted to make a reality through my own hard work and belief in myself. The three hours it took to create the board were probably among the best I had spent in a long, long time. I loved every second of creating that vision board – it felt as if my passion was really coming to fruition right there and then. I even framed it, and put it up where it would be the first thing I saw when I woke up every morning.

How wonderful would it be for you to wake up with something so positive staring right back at you? With your passion, your goals, your inspiration telling you, 'Yes, you can! Now get up and do it'!

Remember, the idea behind your vision board is to remind yourself of who you want to become, what you *really* want to do, the things that you are grateful for and the things along the way that will help you achieve your dreams.

So what will you need to create your very own and totally inspirational vision board? Well, the good news is – not too much!

SELF-CARE ACTION: Create your vision board

- Grab some scissors, glue, a large piece of cardboard – as big as you like – and some magazines (or you can go online and find some images – Pinterest is very good for this).
- Next, write down a word or a sentence that sums up your passion. If you are not sure what your passion

is yet, maybe just write the word 'inspiration', or 'what I love' or 'I've got this', so that you are at least starting to fuel that fire deep within you with things that inspire you.

- Now cut and paste images, words, phrases and colours of the things that you love, that inspire you, that make you feel good inside and that make you really, truly and genuinely smile – because this is your personal masterpiece!

Each and every time you pass by your vision board, visualise that passion coming true. Feel that tingly sensation when you see it come to life. And throughout this month, seek out those very significant others in your life – people you really trust – and tell them about your passion. When you talk about your passion, you are giving it power, and the more you do this, the more you are essentially holding yourself accountable for making sure that it really does come true. Sharing your passions with others allows you to continue to think about how and what you need to do to realise them.

Be aware, however, that once you begin to share your passion with others, you will, of course, meet the pessimists, the cynics. Everyone will have an opinion. I say, surround yourself with the positive people, those who will cheer you on and lift you up – the ones who believe in you. They are the people with dreams and passions, just like you. Together, you will build each other up. Stick with those who say, 'Heck, yes! You can and will do it and I can't wait to see it all unfold.'

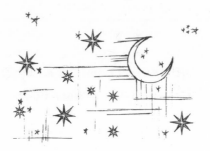

Do Your Research

To make it all happen, research the paths you need to take to get there, the education you might need: the help, the advice, the motivation, the tools, the people, the books, the podcasts, the workshops, the courses. Then put together a plan – one with a timeline and achievable and realistic time-sensitive goals ... because the world is waiting for your passion to come alive.

Month Seven

Shining Your Authentic Light and Finding Your Truth

Our deepest fear is not that we are inadequate.
Our deepest fear is that we are powerful beyond
measure. It is our light not our darkness that
most frightens us.

MARIANNE WILLIAMSON

Think of the best version of yourself as the most authentic version that you can be – the person you are when no one else is around; the person deep within you who desperately wants to come out. Remember her? You feel happiest when you are that person. When you are truly the real you. However, you probably find that this person rarely emerges because of people, situations and life experiences that have made you who you are today.

Have you ever thought that you sound or act like your

mum? Or have you ever been in a situation where you feel you have to be someone else, act in a certain way and, basically, pretend to be someone you are not? This is normal, but it is not positive in the long run because you will start to resent the other person (or people) you are morphing into in order to please others. This is happening because you feel, or someone has told you or society has dictated, that you have to be someone else in order to fit in. And I guarantee you will soon become exhausted trying to be someone you are not in order to please others.

Masking Our Authentic Selves

Before we can look at how to nurture our real, true, authentic selves, we must take a hard look at the masks we wear and when and why we wear them. Why are we so afraid to be our authentic selves?

Throughout our lives, we encounter different people, situations and experiences where we feel we have to be someone else in order to fit in or meet the expectations of those around us. In fact, we wear many of these 'masks' in the course of a day. There is the work mask, the partner mask, the friend mask, the fun mask, the cool mask, the parent mask, the pretty mask and so on. When we wear these masks, we are hiding from our authentic selves. Often we are too afraid to expose who we really are because we fear being mocked and rejected. We worry that we will be deemed 'weird', or 'not lovable', or 'crazy', or 'not good enough', or 'not pretty enough' – you get the point: we are afraid that we will be negatively branded or perceived in a bad light. So we allow ourselves to be someone other than who we really are because that is the safer option. Or so we think.

I used to wear a mask every second of every day. I wore a mask first thing in the morning around my kids. Then at the school gates, I wore the 'I-am-the-best-mum-ever' mask; in my fitness classes, I wore the 'I-can-do-everything-and-my-outfit-looks-great' mask; for work there was the 'I-am-super-smart-I-am-never-wrong-and-always-in-a-good-mood' mask. And if I was having lunch or dinner with my so-called friends, I would wear the 'My-life-is-absolutely-perfect' mask.

Wearing these masks every day, disguising who I really was, became exhausting. I began to resent it. I started to question why I always had to wear them. Why couldn't I just be me? Being someone I thought everyone else wanted me to be really started to wear me down, and it became easy to forget who I truly was, deep down. It was like having to change clothes ten times a day, making sure the outfits were all perfectly matched.

I felt numb and totally out of touch with others. And, if I am honest, completely detached from my own life. What *was* my own life? Did I even have one?

Sometimes we are so used to wearing masks that we forget we are even wearing them. They become so ingrained, such a part of us, that we think we are these people – that our true, authentic selves are the masks we wear. Well, I am here to tell you they are not.

As I discovered through my own self-care journey, in order to start living an authentic life, we have to look hard at the masks we wear and, more importantly, why we feel we have to wear them at all.

So what can we do to shed those masks for good and make ourselves beam with authenticity? This is what we are striving for this month: you are going to make it a habit to be the true, what-you-see-is-what-you-get, 100 per cent amazing you!

The Characteristics of Authentic People

Authentic people are completely comfortable with who they are, even if others may think of them as 'out of the ordinary'. They are true to themselves, and never ever feel the need to wear a mask of any kind. Let's have a look at their make-up:

- They will poke fun at their own imperfections and never, ever try to be perfect. They understand that perfect simply does not exist.
- They enjoy being by themselves because that is when

they are able to do the things they love. There is no fear of having to be seen and no fear of missing out.

- Authentic people love to listen and even see points of views from others' perspectives.
- They will likely have friends from a wide range of different backgrounds.
- They are honest with their feelings, opinions and views and they are willing to talk rationally and calmly about why they feel the way they do.
- They understand and accept that everyone is wired differently, and that is what makes each of us unique.
- If they do not like a situation or conversation or person, then they do not try to fit in, they stay quiet. Simply put, they don't gossip or put anyone down.
- Authentic folks are happy to look back and accept their past and the choices they made rather than make excuses or, worse yet, blame others for their past, lie about it or regret it. The past is what has helped shape them into who they are today.
- Truly authentic people will encourage and support others to just be themselves, and they never look at superficial beauty – they are attracted to what is inside a person rather than what is on the outside.
- Authentic people are slow to pass judgement and understand that every action causes a reaction.
- They have an infectious energy, compassion towards

others and they listen to and respect other people's
opinions and advice (even if they do not agree).

- When they are in the company of others, they rarely
  look at their phones – they choose instead to live in
  the present moment.
- And here's a big one: authentic people understand
  that being authentic is not the same as being 'nice'
  all the time.

SELF-CARE ACTION: Taking off your mask

- List the masks you wear in your life, with whom and
  in which situations. For example, 'I wear the my-life-
  is-perfect mask with X because she always tells me
  how amazing her life is, so I feel I should do the same
  or else she won't like me'.

- Ask yourself if striving to be a certain person and
  living inside your 'masked' world makes you happy.

- Next, write down a list of people who allow you to
  feel 100 per cent you. One of the most fantastic ways
  to reconnect with your authentic self is to surround
  yourself with those people who remind you who you

truly are and who value who you are – people you can tell anything to, including how you feel.

Many of us grew up hearing that we should just be ourselves, and that we could pursue any and all of our dreams, no matter what. And we may tell our children the exact same thing. Yet, as adults, we are often pressured to conform to what others – and society – want us to be, and this is when we lose our authentic selves. But remember, your authentic self is still there; it may just be hidden behind several masks.

How To Shine Your Authentic Light

This month is all about connecting to or rediscovering your true, real self, but how do you go about shining your authentic light?

Embrace being alone

Start by giving yourself space. As I've said, the majority of authentic people embrace being alone. They love having space for themselves. We are constantly around people and activity: our families, co-workers, social engagements, digital devices, etc., so it is easy to be occupied all the time. But what we really all need, every now and then, is some space to breathe.

I find it very strange that in our busy lives we do not make spending time with ourselves a priority. We live in this hectic world that makes us believe that when we are not doing something, we are lagging behind or that everyone else is faster and better than us. If we persist with that mindset and continue believing we must keep up with the Joneses, then we are setting ourselves up for an unhappy life. We will be living in everyone else's shadows, rather than coming out from our own shadow to shine our light.

Just as we put in the time and energy to connect with those we truly care about and love – the relationships that make up our inner circle – we need to do the same with ourselves. We can't turn our lights on if our batteries are not charged. And we can recharge them by simply spending time with ourselves. But how long does that require? All it takes is ten minutes a day. That's it!

SELF-CARE ACTION: Me time

This month, let's create the habit of spending ten minutes a day with ourselves. It might mean simply sitting in silence, and that's great! Or perhaps it's grabbing a green juice and walking to the park or walking around the block a few times. Set your alarm each day as a reminder to take those ten minutes to recharge your batteries. You will be amazed at the wonderful thoughts, inspirations and ideas that can appear as you do so.

List some of the things you're going to do with your ten minutes to yourself each day this month:

When you do give yourself space to recharge, you start to hear what it is you really need and want. You are freed from worrying about, taking care of and giving your energy to everyone else. You get to finally listen to *you* and think without distraction, and you can acknowledge your feelings, rather than shoving them aside. The more you start to listen to yourself, the more real and authentic you become. You start to live your life from a place that is real, rather than the pretend world you are in when wearing all of your masks.

Once you start to feel more connected to your authentic self, you can truly start to hear and feel your gut! And remember, the gut is considered to be the second brain. So when you start to truly listen to your gut, you will understand how you can step out into your life as your authentic self every single day. The connection you have with yourself becomes so much stronger and, of course, real, that you can't imagine living any other way. The masks will fall away once and for all.

When I stopped caring about what other people thought of me and started to truly be me – the real, authentic me – I saw huge improvements in my relationships with other people and in my relationship with myself.

Exercises in Authenticity

As you now know, I am obsessed with yoga and its many, many benefits. If you have done it before, you will know that one of the main components of a yoga practice is the breathing.

In my yoga classes there is a strong emphasis on diaphragmatic breathing, also known as abdominal or belly breathing. It is done by contracting the diaphragm, and I consider it to be one of the most effective breathing techniques. When you do it, air enters the lungs and your belly will expand. This specific exercise is incredibly useful for lowering blood pressure, releasing serotonin (the so-called happy hormone), improving sleep quality and balancing stress hormones. We used this breathing exercise in Month Two, so you should have already formed a healthy habit using it to help you manage stress.

There are also several other breathing exercises that

can be used to boost health and happiness and an overall sense of balance. A large part of our day, if not all of it, is spent breathing involuntarily – our body breathes for us, meaning our breath is not controlled by us. But when we breathe consciously – paying 100 per cent attention to the breath – it is an opportunity for us to connect with ourselves. Simply put, it is an extremely powerful way to get back to our true, authentic selves and this helps to strengthen our physical, mental and emotional well-being.

Alternate-nostril breathing is a great way to do this as it is believed to synchronise the different sides of the brain, creating harmony between the two and getting you back to your true, authentic self. And, of course, this super-powerful breathing exercise has other benefits too. First, it can enhance your respiratory function, increasing the power and endurance of your lungs. Second, it will activate the parasympathetic nervous system (see page 50), which can lower blood pressure. This type of breathing also has the potential to improve your focus and attention span, as well as improving co-ordination.

SELF-CARE ACTION: Alternate-nostril breathing

- Begin by sitting on your yoga mat or cushion on the floor in a comfortable position. Breathe normally for a few moments until you feel yourself become calmer and more present in this moment.
- Rest your left hand in your lap or on your left knee. The index and middle fingers of your right hand should rest on the bridge of your nose and your thumb can be placed over your right nostril. Your ring finger and your little finger can then come to rest on your left nostril.
- With your eyes closed, use your thumb to close your right nostril as you begin the process of inhaling deeply in through your left nostril. Once you have taken a deep breath in, release your thumb and use your little finger to gently close your left nostril. You can then breathe deeply out through your right nostril. Keeping your right nostril open, inhale deeply again and then close your right nostril as you open the left nostril to exhale deeply.
- You have now completed one round and it is a good idea to continue doing so for a few minutes. I personally try to do ten rounds. Remember, one full round is inhaling through both left and right nostrils.

Authenticity Requires Honesty

There are many reasons why we sometimes find it hard to say what we truly feel, so we wear a mask to say them. Or we remain silent because we are too afraid to voice the truth. But we must be honest with ourselves, and with others, or we will continue to live inauthentic lives. We must learn to speak what we truly feel in a loving, kind way.

Conversations with certain people can often seem terrifying. Emotions can be running high, personality differences can manifest or it may just be a super-sensitive topic. However, when you learn to speak your authentic truth without letting emotions get out of hand – staying calm, cool and collected – you will soon find that this leads to more meaningful relationships. You are being honest, you are not hiding anything. The masks are off. And you are shining your true, authentic light.

Tips to Recharge

Every time you are in a situation where you feel you are slipping the mask back on, put these tips into practice:

- **Begin with honesty** Basing everything you say on honest intentions is, in my view, the *number-one* key to authenticity. And yes, I am even talking about stopping those little white lies, too. They may seem harmless, and perhaps they are, but do they make you feel good? Probably not. The truth can be hard to express at first and it can hurt both you and others – but, trust me, dishonesty hurts everyone so much more. Once you start embracing the habit of being honest, with yourself and with others, those feelings of shame, guilt and embarrassment start to fade, once and for all.

- **Start with positive intentions** Begin every conversation and interaction with positive intentions and try to hold on to this positivity, regardless of the direction things go in. If you know you need to have a difficult chat or are entering into a situation where there is a lot of negative energy flowing, take a few breaths before entering the space and say to yourself, 'I am going to bring my positive energy in and keep shining my light'. Then, no matter how difficult things are, you will notice that you are less prone to defensive or angry responses.

- **Acknowledge your role** When communicating with another person, or a group of people, always be aware of what your role is. Are you the listener or the advisor? If your past behaviour or actions are the reason for a conversation that is taking place, be honest about all that has happened (in other words, go back to the first tip) and focus on reaching a resolution. I know this can be hard, but playing the blame game does not do anyone any good at all. This is especially the case if you know that the fault lies with you! Vulnerability is a strength, not a weakness. From vulnerability comes respect. Plus, it is so much easier to move on when you hold yourself accountable.

- **Speak for yourself** Yours is the only truth that you can genuinely, authentically speak, so make sure that you never try to be the voice for anyone else, unless they ask you to be. When you talk to other people, always try to speak from your own perspective and be clear that the opinions and feelings you are offering are your own.

- **Avoid misinterpreting facts** If you do not understand something, that is normal and it is OK. It is when we make our own assumptions about events that we have been told, heard or read – or perhaps even situations that we have experienced – that things start to go wrong. This can often lead to unnecessary negative energy, but also we get labelled as a gossip, and that is just another mask. Observe situations with accuracy and remember that you never know what other people might be going through.

- **Express your emotions** Living an authentic life means never lying about the way you feel, and acknowledging that all of your thoughts, feelings and emotions are valid in any situation. Expressing these emotions, and communicating clearly and calmly with those around you can help you to process and understand them better, as well as helping you to build more meaningful relationships.

Month Eight

Mastering Your Inner Critic

Be careful how you are talking to
yourself because you are listening.

LISA M. HAYES

We all have that little voice inside our head that makes
us doubt ourselves. But sometimes that voice isn't so little!
It can be loud, relentless and deflating. It says things like,
'You're not good enough/pretty enough/clever enough/
successful enough/skinny enough ... ' Or worse: 'You're
terrible at this/you're an embarrassment/you're stupid/
no one likes you/you were only invited out of guilt/you
are ugly/you are fat/no one should waste their time with
you ... '

Sound familiar? Say hello to your mean inner critic –
your own worst enemy. That cruel voice inside of you that
makes you doubt yourself can be a difficult one to silence,

especially if you have spent a long time listening to its criticism and have never questioned it.

It can often seem as though this voice has a negative opinion on just about everything that you do. And, even though you may know that it's not the most reasonable voice to listen to, it will often be the loudest and, therefore, pretty difficult to ignore.

Your inner critic knows your insecurities and will play

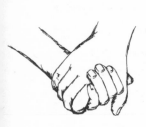

off these self-doubts in order to hold you back. Naturally this will have a detrimental effect on your mood, not to mention your mental health. And, with its relentless intensity, this voice can easily quash your beliefs about your own abilities.

Controlling Your Inner Critic

This month you are going to befriend your inner critic. You're going to assert that you're the boss and tell it to either shape up or ship out because there is a new you in town and you are here to stay.

You are, in the simplest terms, your inner critic's owner. You are in charge. You get to tell it what to say and not the other way around. But, unfortunately, you – as do we all – mostly listen to it when it's putting you down, sometimes even repeating its observations out loud – and worse, starting to believe them! When this happens, you become despondent, demotivated and even depressed. Yet your true, authentic self wants you to be motivated, inspired, passionate and happy.

So having established who your inner critic is – i.e. you – you need to take a long, hard look at why it can spin out of control.

Are You Encouraging Your Inner Critic?

We all compare ourselves to others – their successes, their appearance (inside and out), the 'toys' they have, how much money they have, their 'perfect' relationships, 'perfect' children, 'perfect' homes and, well, their seemingly 'perfect' lives. When it comes to our inner critic, this is the worst thing we can do.

I am here to tell you that a) no one is perfect and b) if they pretend that their life is 'perfect', that is even more reason to believe that it is not.

Fuelled by Social Media

Social media allow us to compare ourselves to others 24/7 (cue Month Three: Digital Detox). But let's be honest, most people are not going to post a photo of themselves when they are having the worst day and suffering from a range of negative emotions because the last thing they want is to let everyone on their feed know how they're feeling.

I don't share all the 'yuck' stuff either. This is because during those times, I am processing: I am working on myself, and I need some alone time. We tend to share those snapshots when life is looking pretty good. But that's just what they are – snapshots of someone's life, rather than a true reflection of their life, all day, every day. Otherwise, you would see the lows along with the highs. So anytime your inner critic rears its head and tries to compare you to someone else, remind yourself that what you are seeing is a snapshot, and that is all it is.

Keeping You Questioning

Not only does your inner critic tell you that so and so is better than you, and that their life is 'perfect', it also works to keep you worrying, ensuring you are never comfortable with who you are:

- Do I look OK?
- Do I fit in?
- Do they honestly want to be friends with me?
- Does he or she truly like me?
- Am I going to get fired?
- Am I doing this right?
- Is everyone looking at me and judging me?

You get it, right? And, in the case of my own inner critic, it drastically over-emphasises what can go wrong. Before I taught myself how to turn down the volume on my inner critic, I would always assume the worst – even when I knew the worst-case scenario was totally unrealistic. If someone cancelled plans with me, I would assume there was an issue with our relationship, or that I had upset them in some way. Also, if something – anything – went wrong during the day, I would immediately blame myself for not having tried hard enough or not being 'good enough'. Sound familiar? Deep down inside we know that these thoughts are irrational, but they still have power over us.

The inner critic plants irrational thoughts in your mind – for example, 'Why were you invited? No one really likes you'. Then it reinforces its power over you with a follow-up along the lines of: 'Look over there – she was invited and she is totally confident. You should be like her. No wonder no one is talking to you!' So the inner critic puts you down and then basically shames you for having had the thoughts it put there in the first place!

Origins of the Inner Critic

The inner critic probably takes a lot of its inspiration from people in your life. It can be an echo of people from your past, or those who are present in your life now. They can be friends, parents, siblings, co-workers or bosses who have said some hurtful things in the past, or even looked at you in a certain way. And this is how your inner critic grows in size and in volume. You may find that it feeds on the negativity and criticism that you absorb from other people.

If someone is persistently putting you down, then you will start to doubt yourself. And that little voice is going to use these criticisms and perpetuate them. So it is a good idea to limit your contact, create boundaries or maybe even disconnect entirely from those negative influences and energy vampires. Once you recognise that your inner critic is not something that you have to pay attention to, it becomes much easier to move forward and take the risks you have always wanted to take.

Tactics of the inner critic
Here are five ways that your personal inner critic will try to damage you:

1. Voicing criticism
When you are thinking about making a change – big or small – or you are trying something new, you might feel both nervous and excited at the same time. For example, when you are trying to achieve your goals, your positive feelings about them may well be drowned out by your mean inner critic. This voice will tell you that you can't possibly succeed and that perhaps it is safer and better for all involved if you do not try at all. Starting today, you are going to remember that this voice is simply self-doubt making an appearance, and that you certainly do not have to listen to it.

2. Discouraging positive action

Your inner critic will often mask itself as the most 'reasonable' option when you are faced with making a decision. It tries very hard to silence your gut feeling, and it will often discourage you in seemingly justifiable ways in order to stop you dead in your tracks and prevent you moving forwards in life. Even though it can seem the *safest* option to listen to your inner critic, you should remember that's not always the *best* one for you and your future. As the great American philanthropist Harry Gray said, 'No one ever achieved greatness by playing it safe.' And we are all worthy of greatness.

3. Making you feel unprepared

Your inner critic loves to criticise your skills, talents, gifts, uniqueness and life experiences. No matter how good you know you are at doing something, this voice always wants you to think that you are not good enough. It will try to damage your self-confidence by insisting that you are simply not ready – and nor will you ever be.

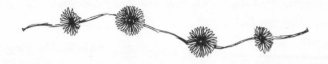

4. Planting body-image doubts

Your inner critic can be harsh and incredibly hurtful. It is certainly not uncommon to dislike aspects of your own appearance (I wish I had thicker hair), but your inner critic thrives on this insecurity bigtime. Any slight negative thoughts you have about your body, such as your weight or signs of ageing, can quickly become the main focus of your inner critic. And, once you give this negative voice within you the power it's looking for, body-image issues can be incredibly hard to overcome.

5. Irrational persistence

One of the most powerful ways that your inner critic will attack you is through an irrational persistence of the negative message that it wants to get across. This voice will often rehash the same criticisms over and over again, like an old stuck record. Do you really want to listen to that over and over again for the rest of your life? No way!

Silencing Your Inner Critic

It is important to make these steps a habit so that each time your inner critic tries to rear its head, your healthy habits immediately kick in. Then it will eventually lose its voice, once and for all.

SELF-CARE ACTION: Question your inner critic

First and foremost, you need to question why your inner critic is focusing on certain things. Perhaps it speaks the loudest when you are thinking about changing careers or embarking upon a new healthy-eating plan. This voice might attempt to deter you by making you feel as if you are only going to fail anyway, so why try?

Write down three things that you are most afraid of failing at, or are afraid to start doing.

Now write down any negative thoughts associated with the three sentences above. What you write here is your inner critic making an appearance.

Now write down what you, your authentic self, have to say. Write down at least three positive thoughts associated with those three things you are most afraid of failing at or of doing.

Anytime your inner critic starts up with those negative thoughts, you now have the ammunition to shoot it back down.

Yes, your inner critic can be loud, persistent and discouraging, but it is just one voice among many. If you have positive feelings about something, never allow this one lone voice to have the final say.

SELF-CARE ACTION: Answer back

Always answer back. Yup, that's right, you get the last word. One of the reasons why the inner critic is able to throw you off course is that you are often unable or unwilling to fight back. So every time a negative thought surfaces from your inner critic, refute it with a positive one: when the inner critic says, 'You're a failure', you respond with, 'I'm a success'; when you hear, 'You're not good enough', you respond with, 'I am enough'. You will soon find that this voice starts to back down in the face of reason.

Write down your inner critic's most common and loudest negative statements about you. Then, next to each one, turn that statement on its head. For example, if my inner critic says, 'You fail at everything', I write, 'My failures give me an opportunity to learn and grow in order to achieve success'.

SELF-CARE ACTION: Be kind

If you are not giving yourself the love and positive attention that you deserve, then of course your inner critic is going to take hold. Negativity thrives where it already has a foothold.

You do not have to wait for this voice to pipe up to give yourself a dose of kindness, and you should do so several times a day. Remind yourself of the things that others like about you. These moments of kindness to others and to yourself are the things that define you; they are the *real* you, not those brief moments of negative energy from deep within.

Write down as many kind words as you can think of that people have said to you and about you:

Being able to take control back from your inner critic for good might seem out of reach, but when you take the time to nurture yourself, understand your thought processes and make a habit of doing so, trust me, you will win. And win big! Once you make this healthy habit your own, you will be able to make decisions with much more confidence and grab all of the amazing opportunities that come your way in life without second-guessing yourself.

Opposition Thinking

A good exercise to practise every day this month to help control your inner critic is called 'opposition thinking'.

You may often dismiss your thoughts as being insignificant but – and this is a *big* but – your thoughts are the driving force behind your feelings, your beliefs and the path you take through life.

To begin with let's examine our thoughts in a little more detail. Some of them will hold more weight than others. This will likely be because they seem more plausible or rational, and therefore urge you to take action and make decisions. On the other hand, some thoughts will be fleeting and quickly forgotten. If you are anything like me, you may find it difficult to manage your thoughts, and that is totally normal! However, in my experience, when my thoughts are all over the place, it is usually because I've allowed those negative thoughts to stay present in my mind for too long, causing me to believe that they are justified. It usually starts with one negative thought, which then causes other negative thoughts to spiral out of control. To put it simply, negative thoughts breed more negative thoughts.

When negative thoughts remain in your mind your mood is going to be adversely affected, your self-esteem can become damaged and you may even notice that your energy levels are lowered, as you are drained by negativity. It can even affect how much enjoyment you take from the things that you usually find very pleasurable.

When you truly start to acknowledge that everything in your life can be influenced by your thoughts, you are taking a giant leap towards mastering that inner critic. Learning how to manage your thoughts will better equip you to maintain a positive mindset with positive thoughts, and this will have a knock-on effect on how you view yourself, how you treat yourself and also how you interact with those around you.

Opposition thinking is an incredibly powerful tool when it comes to managing your thoughts and we are going to use it this month to help us create that healthy habit of positive thinking. It is super-simple, but you must commit to doing it. You may find you have to force yourself to really embrace this concept at first, but it will soon become second nature and will, in no time, start to silence that inner critic.

SELF-CARE ACTION:
Opposition thinking exercise

The rule is that every time you have a negative thought, you have to replace it with the opposite thought – but you must do so as soon as the negative thought enters your mind.

For example, if you are thinking that you have failed at something that you tried to do during your day, then you immediately replace this thought by saying to yourself that you tried your hardest to do something difficult, that you learned from it and will get it right next time. If you are saying you are not good enough, follow it up with 'I am good enough'. You need to repeat these positive thoughts at least three times, and you can even say them out loud. I find that actually vocalising them pushes me to believe that they are true.

List your most common negative thoughts here – the stuck record, on-repeat thoughts. Next to them, write the opposite, positive one, making sure you write it down three times:

So, just to re-iterate, throughout this month, when you wake in the morning, go to bed at night or when you are simply having a tough day, I want you to write down whatever negative thought came into your head. Write the opposite, the positive statement, and discount that negative thought three times! Once you have written it down, then repeat it to yourself, either out loud or mentally, three times. So the next time you hear that negative thought rear its head, you can shoot it back down.

That way you'll be on your way to finally saying good-bye to your inner critic.

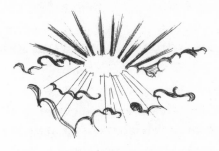

Month Nine

Learning to Love Yourself

As I began to love myself I freed myself
of anything that is no good for my health –
food, people, things, situations, and
everything that drew me down and
away from myself. At first I called this
attitude a healthy egoism. Today
I know it is 'Love of Oneself'.

CHARLIE CHAPLIN

Self-love. It truly is the new buzzword these days – the
kale of the self-care world. And, frankly, I think it is here
to stay. I remember listening to Kris Carr, best-selling
author of *Crazy Sexy You*, and laughing out loud when
she said, 'Remember when kale was just kale, before it
got a publicist!' Well, it is the same with self-love. It got
a publicist, and it is now the talk of the town. However,

most people still don't have a clue as to what self-love truly means.

As we learned last month, the last thing we want to do is leave our self-worth in the hands of our inner critic, or anyone else for that matter! Constantly seeking the love of everyone else is exhausting, but by learning to love ourselves we can finally stop playing the victim.

How Do You Love Yourself?

I often ask my students if they truly love themselves and most of the time, they say, 'Yes!' I then follow it up with this question: 'How do you show yourself that you love yourself?' The most common responses are, 'I go to yoga', 'I get a lot of massages', 'I get my nails done', 'I have a spa day', 'I take candlelit baths' or, 'I meditate'. Yes, these are all a form of self-care. You are taking care of yourself physically, but where is the emotional part? That is the self-love piece of the puzzle that many of us are missing.

A good way to understand this is to think back to when you were a child and remember what you needed to feel loved. Did you prefer to have the toy you wanted or the hug that you needed? When you were upset, did you need a cookie or someone to take care of you? You wanted a hug and needed someone to take care of you, right? That is love. And, self-love is no different. We have to hug ourselves often – every single day – when we have done something fantastic or when we feel down in the dumps.

We need to take care of ourselves. We
need to love ourselves as much as we hug,
take care of and love everyone else in
our lives.

Be Your Own Cheerleader

I know that self-love is often the hardest
kind of love. As we have learned in the
previous months, it is easier for us to
focus on our flaws, our mistakes and our
failures. But we need to become our own
cheerleaders – we can't expect others to do
it for us.

I was captain of my cheerleading squad in
high school. No matter what, even if we were
losing and there was absolutely no way we could make a
comeback and win, I had a job to do and that was to cheer
the team on and keep the crowd in good spirits!

Since then, I have become my own cheerleader. I
cheer myself on. I need all of me to work together, to
love myself in order to get through the hard times. So
how about looking at yourself as a wonderful, amazing,
incredible, super-talented team? Sometimes you win and
sometimes you lose, but find your inner cheerleader and
let it speak to your emotions and feelings, and tell them,
'Hey, it's all going to be OK!' Let it tell your body parts
to 'Keep going': your muscles, 'Yes, you can do this',

your cells to 'Keep working together, guys', your head to 'Stay focused', your heart that 'It's OK to feel because you're going to get through this', your gut to 'Start listening up' and your spirit to 'Keep moving forwards!' Now *that* is self-love at its best and you can achieve that this month.

Those Who Focus On Self-Love

When we are armed with self-love, we feel braver, empowered, worthy, and we don't feel like we need to audition for the love and attention of others in order to fill any gaps in our self-love. This month we are going to start a self-love practice that is fun and easy to incorporate into our daily lives. But first, let's look at what it is that people who truly love themselves do differently from those of us who don't.

Do any of these statements sound familiar?

- When I get that promotion, then I'll be happy.
- When I find the right person to marry, then I'll be happy.
- When I lose ten pounds, then I'll be happy.

People who love themselves don't put such conditions on their love for themselves. They don't wait until everything is perfect to finally say, 'Oh, X, Y and Z just happened. So now I'm allowed to love myself and my life'. People who love themselves practise loving themselves in the moment. For example, they say, 'OK, I didn't get that promotion, but that means it probably wasn't right for me and something better is on its way'; or, 'That relationship didn't work out for reasons that maybe I don't know about or understand now, but I know that someone better is waiting for me'; or, 'It's not about how much weight I lose, that's just a number. I am taking care of myself and that's the most important thing'.

People who love themselves do not have huge egos. I'm sure you have come across people who act like they have everything. They are arrogant and make everyone around them feel as if they are 'less than'. Now remember – and try hard to remember this because you will keep coming across these types of people, over and over again – these egocentric people are just hurting. Usually, they are insecure and crying out for love.

People who love themselves are not selfish. When we truly love ourselves, we become self-less! Self-love makes you a better parent, friend, co-worker, sibling and so on. People who love themselves don't put their own needs first if it means sacrificing the needs of others. But they do set boundaries and know when to say no. They are compassionate and understanding, but they will not be taken advantage of, nor will they spend too much time – or any time at all – with those who take, take, take (aka energy vampires).

Self-loving people know what they want out of their

relationships with others. They know that respect goes both ways, and if their boundaries are repeatedly crossed, then they have the guts to walk away for good. However, self-loving people will admit when they are wrong, and they certainly don't apportion blame. In fact, they expect to be wrong at times and take responsibility for their mistakes. This is because self-loving people know that they are always learning from their mistakes, and that mistakes lead to future successes.

And lastly, self-loving people don't shove their emotions under a rug and leave them hidden. Nor do they let loose in an unhealthy way. Instead, they accept each emotion as is, and try to understand why they are feeling it in a constructive and reasonable way.

Self-love, well, it's hard! But if we don't start to love ourselves as the wonderful people we are, we will be unhappy with every aspect of our lives. We have to learn to love ourselves *unconditionally*, starting today.

Accept Yourself to Love Yourself

Self-love can seem incredibly difficult to put into practice. It is about accepting our current condition as it stands today – good or bad – and saying, 'I love me'. When you love yourself, you can get through anything. But, like all journeys, learning to love yourself begins with small steps.

Loving yourself means becoming fully present with

your feelings, your needs, your wants. It means having compassion for yourself. You can do this by creating some loving habits for yourself, beginning with accept-ance: acceptance of the past, the people who might have helped shape who you are today and your life experi-ences – good and bad. If you hide your acceptance of yourself, then it shows others – and you – that you are ashamed of who you are and, therefore, can't truly love yourself.

Acceptance is being willing to accept *all* of you, to love *all* of you; it is accepting that you can't change the past or predict the future. It is when you finally learn to stop judging yourself and start loving yourself instead.

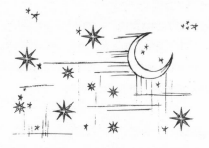

When you start to love yourself, you start to accept that negative experiences are an inevitable part of life, and that we are all born with the strength to overcome them. You understand that dwelling on pain and suffering does not serve you – that it only results in more pain and suffering. It is OK to feel pain, and it is OK to ask for support in order to overcome this pain. Every one of your feelings is valid and it is OK to express them to those around you. It is OK to fail. It is OK to succeed. It is OK to be disappointed. But it is also OK to be proud of all that you have achieved. You can be strong, you can be weak, you can be sad, you can be happy. And you certainly don't have to meet anyone else's expectations in order to be a complete human being. Self-love is born of the acceptance of your flaws, your hopes, your authenticity and your faith that you are perfect just the way you are. Make a promise to yourself to stop hiding from yourself, and from others, and to start loving yourself as you are today.

Set Your Intention For the Day

Starting this month, I want you to set an intention each and every morning before you get out of bed. Make a deliberate effort to create the day you want to have. Here are some things to consider:

- How do you want to feel today?
- What do you want to happen today?
- What decisions can you make today that are right for you?
- What healthy food do you want to nourish yourself with today?
- What exercise can you do today to show your body how much you love all that it does for you?

Remember, you are intending to have an amazing day and to love yourself. It might not turn out that way, but you are putting it out there; you are going into the day with a super-positive, happy attitude, and doing the things that make you feel good about yourself.

SELF-CARE ACTION:
Create your intention

Get into the habit of loving yourself and all that you do. Then encapsulate it in one sentence. Some good examples are:

- Today I will love myself.
- I love my body for all that it does for me.
- I am always doing the best I know how.
- I let go of negative self-talk.
- I am learning and growing each and every day.

Write your intention here:

Remind yourself of your intention throughout your day and put it into action. When we put our intentions into action, we are more likely to start believing them to be true.

Mental and Physical Dieting

We are going to go on two diets this month. Remember, the definition of diet here is a lifestyle and *not* some regime designed to starve the body, mind or spirit. We are going on a loving diet, both mentally and physically.

SELF-CARE ACTION:
Your mental and physical 'diet'

First up, the mental diet. Each day this month for ten minutes, listen to or read something uplifting: a podcast on self-love, a few songs that make you feel good about yourself or a chapter of an inspiring book. Just make sure you do something every day this month to fill your mind with love because what we focus on becomes more real. So by focusing on loving ourselves each and every day this month, we can get closer to that reality.

List your uplifting podcasts, songs and books for the month here:

Next, you're going to upgrade your physical diet. What do I mean by this? Start incorporating the foods that the body loves. Hopefully you created a healthy habit around food in Month One, and now you can go deeper this month. Make a list of the foods that you know make your body feel great. For me, it's green tea – I think I have five to six cups a day of the *best* green tea every single day, and I feel so good after drinking it. I also love a green juice. After drinking a freshly pressed green juice, I always feel fantastic. Additionally, I love my ginormous leafy green salad with lentils, quinoa, pumpkin seeds, red onion, tomatoes, avocado, chia seeds and a simple olive oil, vinegar and lemon juice dressing. I love this salad so much because not only do I know that it is good for me, but I feel great after eating it. Yes, these foods are going to nourish me, but I also feel good about myself knowing that I am feeding my body with pure goodness.

My feel-good foods are

So what foods make you feel good both on the inside and out? List a month's worth of foods that you love (depending on when you are reading this, you will list between twenty-eight and thirty-one different foods that make you feel so, so good):

Your homework this month is to have at least one of these foods every single day. And I bet you will find you have many, many more of them combined. I mean, just think about my ginormous salad!

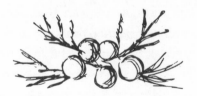

Self-love Actions

Lastly, you are going to create a list of self-loving actions. What have you done each day this month to show yourself some love? A self-loving action could be as simple as:

- making a green juice
- booking a weekend getaway for one
- starting that blog
- starting the book you've always wanted to write
- cooking in the kitchen with your kids or friends
- having a family or friends' movie night
- walking to work
- making a healthy meal
- calling a long-lost friend
- saying sorry
- writing a thank-you note
- creating an uplifting playlist.

SELF-CARE ACTION: Your self-love action list

Make your self-loving action list here:

Take the time this month to become your own best friend. Stop apologising to yourself and to others for just being you. Every morning, step out into the world as yourself. And when you go to bed at night, tell yourself how proud you are of yourself for the accomplishments of that day. Choose to love yourself, because when you do, a whole bunch of wonderful things start to happen!

Month Ten

Say Goodbye to Fear and Hello to Courage

False Evidence Appearing Real

Those who are successful in creating a life that is full of happiness have a particular quality in common: they are courageous. These people go after the things they want and push through the self-doubt, the risks, the scary bits and the fear! This month, we are going to get on track and learn how to do the exact same thing. So say goodbye to fear and hello to courage.

The first thing to realise when it comes to facing our fears is that self-doubt is normal – totally 100 per cent normal. Apart from when fear alerts us to real physical danger, it is simply one of our inner critic's weapons. We now know from Month Eight that we mustn't give that voice any more power than it already has. Remember, you are in control.

And fear? Well, fear is just an illusion, fuelled by the energy we choose to give it. But unfortunately for many of us, we fuel our fear so much that it is constantly chasing after us. Then we try to run away from the fear that is fuelling us! And it's exhausting.

Do you often think: 'I really want to do X, but I am absolutely petrified because I might'

(fill in the blank).

This sentiment is very common and, sadly, holds many of us back from ever realising our full potential or doing the things that we really want to try.

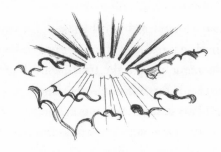

Can We Banish Fear For Ever?

As much as I would like to tell you that you can banish fear for ever, it is still going to appear every so often (just like your inner critic). But you are going to become friends with your fear. It is always going to be there, and the bigger the goal or dream, the bigger the fear. But it's not going to hold you back or control you any more, and you will learn how to use its energy to propel you forwards, to get to a place where you are filled with courage.

There is a quote that I live by (one of many): 'No one ever really fails; they simply just quit'. This is so true. Courage is moving forwards even if there are no guarantees; it is knowing that you can pick yourself up, dust yourself off and keep going.

Face Your Fears

We have to face the fear, understand why we have it in the first place and then befriend it.

I have had a lot of fear in my life: fear of rejection, fear of failure, fear of success, fear of not being good enough, fear of embarrassment, fear of the truth, fear of letting people down, fear of unworthiness ... My relationship with fear caused me to be afraid of doing or achieving anything. When I let it control me, I became insecure, unworthy and scared, preferring to play it safe, rather than take any risks. I have learned, through my own journey, that I will always have fears. But once I started to use them to fuel my intentions, I realised that fear was my friend. Without it, I would not have pursued my yoga career, started a food blog or any of my online businesses or even written this book! Fear was the driving force behind achieving both the small and the big things. And, when that happened, I started to feel empowered, worthy and courageous.

I have found that those who are successful in creating

the life that they love have this in common. They are all courageous. They push through the fear. They use the energy of the fear to go after the things they truly want.

SELF-CARE ACTION:
Identify and overcome your fears

The very first step towards owning and controlling your fears is to identify and understand them. What are you afraid of? What fears are stopping you from taking that risk, that leap of faith?

Being aware of your fears is noticing what it does to your body, your mind and even your spirit. What happens to you when you think about your fears? Do you shut down? Does your inner critic start chatting? Does anxiety begin to kick in? Does your authentic light start to dim? Do you feel stressed? Let's get into how and what you are feeling when fear is alive within you.

Write down some of your most common fears:

Now remember I said that fear is your friend? Well, it is; and having identified your fears, you need to embrace them. Yes, you must hug and even love your fears!

Feelings of fear are there to keep you safe. When you sense any kind of danger – whether that is being chased by a bear, having to give a presentation or arriving at a party knowing no one but the hostess – you feel fear. It is there to protect you from failing, from embarrassment, from criticism.

Fear is built around a scenario you construct – it is based on a story you tell yourself. But is it true or false? Will everyone really laugh at you when you give your presentation? The answer is mostly likely no. And when you walk into that party not knowing a soul, is everyone going to start whispering about you? Again, probably not.

It is up to you to rewrite the story that our fears create. Use the butterflies inside you to drive you to take that risk. Then rewrite the ending: you nail your presentation and everyone claps; you walk into the party confident and with a smile on your face, engaging others in conversation first.

If we never face the fear head-on, give that presentation in front of our colleagues or start to talk to strangers at that party, then fear wins and we don't grow. We stay small. And none of us is here to play it safe and stay small.

In *Daring Greatly: How the Courage to Be Vulnerable Transforms the Way We Live, Love, Parent and Lead*, Brené Brown wrote: 'Being vulnerable is NOT a weakness.' But it was (in my view) widely perceived as such. We fear showing our vulnerable side – our weaknesses and not our strengths – because revealing our vulnerability feels like exposing our naked selves. In fact, all our fears stem from being 'seen', from running the risk of being criticised, of failing, of not being 'perfect', of being 'not enough'. But guess what? People like, in fact they love, *real* people. The second we try to mask our vulnerability, we let fear win. And that's when it becomes our enemy. So we should express our fear, rather than hold it in and pretend everything is hunky dory.

Being vulnerable is a reminder that there is no escape from fear, and that it is OK to feel sad, to be scared, to feel pain. It is also OK to ask for help, to tell others how we feel when we are scared, lonely, worried or angry. When we let the emotions out, fear is no longer in control. Vulnerability is the key to facing our fears. And, once we do that, we can see that we can both fail and succeed, be both weak and strong, sad and happy.

Teddy Roosevelt put the advantages of facing your fears perfectly in his 'Citizenship In A Republic' speech in Paris in 1910:

> *It is not the critic who counts; not the man who points out how the strong man stumbles, or where the doer of deeds could have done them better. The credit belongs to the man who is actually in the arena, whose face is marred by dust and sweat and blood; who strives valiantly; who errs, who comes short again and again, because there is no effort without error and shortcoming; but who does actually strive to do the deeds; who knows great enthusiasms, the great devotions; who spends himself in a worthy cause; who at*

the best knows in the end the triumph of high achievement,
and who at the worst, if he fails, at least fails while daring
greatly, so that his place shall never be with those cold and
timid souls who neither know victory nor defeat.

Controlling Fear and Building Courage

My definition of courage is to act in spite of hardship, challenge, pain, despair and anxiety; to make fear simply the opening act in your journey to discover and live who you authentically are.

No one is 'fearless'. It just happens that some people are better equipped than others to use its energy to move through the scary moments. I mean, nobody ever looked at Everest from basecamp and said, 'Right, I'm not scared and this is going to be a piece of cake'. They got through it by using their fear to fuel them. And as for bravery – well, that is having the ability to truly feel your fear.

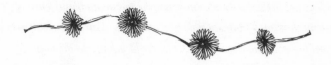

So the real questions are: how do we find the courage within us? And do I have any in the first place? The second question is a rhetorical one because yes, we *all* have courage. Courage is there – in you, too. Let's go back to the first question and figure out how to tap into that courage.

We've already seen that we need to admit to ourselves when we feel fear and not deny it. However, we don't have to create a story around it. We simply accept that we are human and that we have fear. Plain and simple.

It also helps to connect with the greats of our time and those from the past. Recognise that your heroes and role models have also experienced fear. But they didn't focus on the feelings associated with their fear; instead, they focused on what they needed to do about it. Feeling fear means that you are on the verge of growth or a new direction. But you won't grow if you don't take the next step. Whether this step is big or small doesn't matter. You can take baby steps. It's purely about taking the step in the first place.

You can also look at this using the analogy of a yoga pose. What you perceive as small – for example, going a tiny bit deeper into a pose – is, in fact, huge for your body! You might think that moving one millimetre more into a pose than you did last time is nothing to shout about, but if your body could talk, it would tell you how good it feels. It is the same thing with fear and courage. Take a small step towards facing your fears and you'll gain a huge amount of courage!

SELF-CARE ACTION: Use your fears

Are you afraid of:

- public speaking
- rejection

- flying
- heights
- intimacy
- failure
- commitment
- being laughed at
- voicing an opinion?

List your fears here:

Now write down how you can use the energy from these fears and do something about them:

- Do you need to sign up for a public-speaking course?
- Should you get some fear-of-flying therapy?
- Could you sign up for rock climbing at your gym?
- Who can you open up to about your commitment obstacles?
- Who can you open up to about all of your fears?

Get the fears out into the open. Once you recognise what they are, the next time you are faced with them, it will be easier and easier to take those small steps towards courage.

SELF-CARE ACTION: List those you admire

Write down five people you admire, even if they scare you a bit. Ahem, that's your fear knocking, so challenge it with some courage and start to hang around these people a bit more. Or listen to their podcasts more or read more of their books ... Perhaps even invest in a mentor – yes, mentors are wonderful. The point is to be around people who you are inspired by, who motivate you and who strengthen and empower you. They say that we become the average of the five people we spend the most time around. Who are your five?

Never Let Fear Get In the Way of ...

I have five top things that I believe you should never allow your fear to get in the way of. If one or all of these things pops out at you, write down how and maybe with whom you can work through the fear by drawing on your courage.

1. Forgiveness
Forgiveness can be *really* hard, but when you forgive, it heals your relationships with others and with yourself.

Nothing drains your emotional energy quite like holding onto negativity. Holding a grudge is detrimental to you first and foremost, so always try to forgive, and be sure to voice this forgiveness to those who need to hear it.

2. Love
When you approach a new love with reservations because of a past experience, you run the risk of not fully enjoying what is happening in the present moment. Love makes you vulnerable, and you now know that is a strength. Learning to love without fear, and with an open heart and courage, will inevitably enable you to invite an abundance of love into your life through all of your relationships.

3. Ambition
Following your dreams without the fear of failure or judgement from others is the only way to truly fulfil your ambitions. Life is short, so don't waste it doing something that you don't genuinely want to do. Seek your passion (remember Month Six) and follow this path. It is the best way to live an authentic, happy life.

4. Intuition
Listening to your intuition can often be scary, especially if that little voice is telling you to do something difficult, like moving to a new city or taking a new job. But always listen to your heart and don't let the fear of the unknown stop you from having a new adventure.

5. Truth

Always speaking with honest intentions, regardless of the consequences, is the only way to be true to yourself. Holding your thoughts and feelings inside when you want to express them to someone is going to cause frustration to build up – and this isn't good for anybody. So always say what's on your mind, but remember to do so with compassion.

SELF-CARE ACTION: Test your courage

The situations and interactions that you avoid due to fear will, of course, be unique to you. However, a good way to overcome these fears is to deliberately put yourself in these situations. For example, you may have a fear of exercising in public because of what others will think about you. However, you will soon see that when you do exercise in public, no one is in the least bit concerned with what you are doing.

We build up these worries to the point where they become actual fears, but the reality is that they are all in our heads. That isn't to say that they feel any less real, or any less scary, but by pushing ourselves to embrace these situations we can work to overcome these fears.

List the fears you are going to use your courage to confront this month:

Month Eleven

Live with Purpose and Permit Yourself to Change

The two most important days of your life
are the day you are born and the day you
find out what your purpose is.

MARK TWAIN

Hands up if you are so focused on how you're not where you think you should be that you never celebrate how far you have come. We all need to start being OK with where we are today because it will lead us to our purpose. And we all have a purpose here on earth.

Research has shown that living with purpose may lead to a longer life, regardless of how old you are. When I use the term 'living with purpose' I simply mean leading a life that is personally satisfying and fulfilling. This can be down to many factors, but will usually involve embracing your passions, filling your life with love and finding your sources of happiness.

Living your purpose is one of the most amazing things you can do with your life. Of course, it is always easier to just play it safe, or as I like to call it, stay 'stuck'. But Month Eleven is about becoming unstuck. It is about giving yourself permission to change. This gives you the freedom to grow, to experience and to really live. Forcing yourself to stay the same for ever basically kills your life's purpose.

To start the ball rolling, ask yourself the following:

- Are you currently satisfied with your life?
- Do you wake up every morning excited to discover what the day will bring?
- Do you know what fulfils you?

Embrace Your Weird, Wonderful Self

Some people think change is weird. I say, the weirder the better! My kids call me weird and I take it as a compliment. I would rather they said that I am weird than that I'm boring, or dull, or stuck or always the same.

It took me a really long time to get to grips with living with purpose. It's so much easier to go through life with the same routine, the same people, the same everything. But it is certainly not as much fun. For me, having gone through the motions, day after day, month after month, year after year, I got to a certain point and asked: 'Is this it? Surely there must be more to my life?' And the answer is, of course, 'Yes, there is.' But it was up to me to make the change.

I had to become responsible for my own change. No one could change my life for me. I realised that I wanted to leave a legacy. I didn't just want people saying, 'She was a nice girl' – and that's it.

When I started to think about the legacy that I would want to leave, I came to my senses. I realised that I could live with purpose, just like my heroes – the inspirational people in my life (see Month Ten, page 190). What made them any different from me? Absolutely nothing, apart from the fact that they decided to really live!

We simply must live life to its fullest, to make every day as good as we possibly can, so that when we go to bed every night, we can sleep knowing that we really, truly lived. No one can tell you what your life purpose is – I certainly can't; and no one told me what mine was either. Why? Because your life's purpose is unique to you. And that is why some people will think that your choices are weird and that even having a life's purpose is a bit odd. But that is the point. Because of its very uniqueness, only you can express it in your own weird and unique way.

Remember I mentioned the blank stares that Bill Gates and Steve Jobs received early in their careers when discussing what they wanted to do with the technology they were creating? Think how different things would be if they had listened to the sceptics. But they didn't. They listened to their own unique ideas, regardless of what others said, thought or did. And now we are being called on to wake up, smell the coffee and take action!

Of course, it is easy to get distracted or pulled in a different direction because that's life. It is one big roller-coaster ride. But our own unique track is always right there underneath us. It curves, twists and even flips upside down occasionally. But at the end of the day that track is our life's purpose, taking us on the ride of a lifetime. It is up to us if we want to get in the cart and follow the direction that we truly want to go in.

I noticed that when I found my purpose, I felt more alive inside. When we are ready for change, our whole bodies beam with anticipation, the cameras are on and we are ready for action.

Passion and Purpose

When it comes to purpose, we also need passion (see Month Six, 'Finding, Believing in and Building Your Passions'). Passion and purpose co-exist; they hold each other's hands.

You probably know by now

that my passions in life are yoga, healthy eating and self-care. I love to do yoga, I love to eat well, educating myself more and more about wholefoods, and I love to incorporate small moments of self-care into my life. I also love to write about these things and to talk about them with others. I couldn't live my life with purpose without them.

My purpose in life is to make sure that the people I teach, meet and connect with, along with those closest to me, never feel as negatively about themselves as I have felt about myself in the past. There it is. Out in the open. That is what I want my legacy to be. That is my purpose in life.

I know what it is like to be around people who try to bring you down, damage you, shout, scream, walk into a room and to fill it with negative energy, leaving you feeling so bad about yourself that you want to curl up and cry. Yup, been there many times and it didn't stop until I decided to stop being around those people. I want to fill people with joy. I want to talk calmly, kindly, and compassionately to others. I want to listen, lend a shoulder, motivate, inspire, be other people's loudest cheerleader and walk into a room full of people and fill it with positive energy. When I think about that, it makes me feel so good inside – so emotional – that I know it's my purpose.

When I interact with anyone, no matter who they are or what the situation is, I want to walk away knowing that

I might have inspired them. It might mean giving them a hug, a smile, laughter, empathy, compassion – whatever they need. But I always leave hoping that I have somehow made them feel, at the very least, a little bit better about themselves. That is my purpose in life.

Do You Know Your Purpose?

We all need to do some work in order to uncover our purpose. I certainly didn't wake up one morning knowing, with total clarity, exactly what I wanted my purpose in life to be. My purpose was there, but I had to fine-tune it and truly understand what it was I wanted by asking some questions.

Now it is your turn. Spend some time contemplating the questions below. Most likely, you won't be able to answer them in one go. That is totally normal. Take this month to consider them in order to get some more clarity around living with purpose.

Ask yourself:

- Am I currently satisfied with my life?
- Do I wake up every day excited to discover what the day will bring?
- Do the people in my life help me to live with purpose?
- How can I make every day more exciting and fulfilling?

Every single person in the world has a reason and a purpose for being here. Some find it easier than others to know what that purpose is, but within each of us there is a talent and a passion just waiting to be explored, which helps lead us to our purpose. We'll expand on these questions later in this chapter, and look at uncovering your purpose.

Be Inspired by Others

If you know someone who is already living their life having discovered what their unique purpose is, then it can be inspirational to observe them. The happiness that person feels and spreads to those around them is contagious. It is easy to see and it is certainly something that everyone would love to discover for themselves.

Some people tend to find their purpose in life relatively early on. However, this is rare. Many of us walk many, many paths on countless different journeys before knowing the right path to take, and how to navigate it. That was me.

Tips to Challenge Yourself

Overleaf are some ideas to help you figure out what your purpose is, and understand how you can begin to make it a more significant part of your life.

Only by pushing yourself out of your comfort zone and truly seeking your own truth will you be able to shift your perspective and truly open yourself up to the possibility of new experiences.

When you challenge yourself in this way, you allow your authentic self to rise to the surface. Once you have uncovered the changes that you want to make, grab your courage and use the fear to propel you to move forwards (see Month Ten). It will then be easier to visualise how your life could be different and to think about how you will instigate changes.

SELF-CARE ACTION:
Identify your gifts

Paying attention to yourself, the world around you and the things that you are good at will enable you to identify your gifts. When doing this, it is helpful to think back to the moments in your life when you were truly happy. These are likely to be a combination of experiences from your recent past and way back in your childhood.

Once you have a memory in mind, answer these questions:

- What were you doing?

- Who were you doing it with?

- How did you truly feel in this moment?

Try to establish if there are any connections between each of the memories, and pay attention to any particular skills or talents you were using at the time. This will help you to establish common themes that you can then build upon and explore further.

SELF-CARE ACTION:
Meditate on your thoughts

Taking time out from the constant stimulation and chaos of the world is essential for being able to process your thoughts. It is, of course, going to be much harder to see the bigger picture when you are contending with a million other thoughts. This is why meditation is a great tool for getting to the root of your most positive thoughts and better understanding how they can serve you in living with purpose.

Try taking a walk during which you can have a conversation with yourself. Yes, talk to yourself!

The idea here is to create a still and silent setting in which your emotions can be allowed to unfold. Doing so, once a day, is a great way to continuously work to enhance your understanding of your experiences and current situation, and *feel* your feelings – all of which are conducive to learning more about your purpose.

SELF-CARE ACTION: Go beyond the norm

Eleanor Roosevelt once said, 'Do one thing that scares you every day', in the belief that this was a key part of self-discovery. Knowing your comfort zone and making an effort to push yourself out of it will help you to better understand your purpose.

Only when you embrace uncertainty can you really unlock your true potential. Trying different things that challenge your sense of security might not only confirm what you already know about yourself, but also lead you to discover new talents and ideas.

Each day, over the next month, do something that scares you and write about it. For inspiration, start here with your first day then continue in your journal or diary:

SELF-CARE ACTION:
Spread your passion

One of the best things about discovering your passion and purpose in life is being able to share it with others. Making someone else's life a bit brighter by spreading some positivity around is great for everyone involved. It could be one of the most rewarding parts of this path you have decided to embark upon.

You will also notice that when you share yourself with other people in this way, they will be more drawn to sharing themselves and their energy with you as well.

Make a list of people in your life – from friends and family to the newspaper boy and local shop assistant – who you could spread more positivity to.

Taking the First Step

Taking the first step to changing your life can be scary, but it is leading you towards an authentic and exciting existence. Once you have an idea about what it is you want to do – what your purpose in life is – then the time to take a leap of faith and move ahead with your plans has arrived. Remember, it is generally irrational fear that holds you back, and this can be overcome simply by not giving power to those thoughts, and using their energy to propel yourself forwards instead.

QUESTIONNAIRE: Uncovering your unique purpose

Before you answer each of the questions below, breathe in through the nose and out of the mouth three times to help create space between your thoughts. Once you have read a question, close your eyes for a moment or two and listen inwardly for the answer – because the answers are not around you, they are deep *within* you.

- What is my purpose for being alive right here, right now?

- What are my passions in life?

- What do I do that helps others?

- What traits are unique to me?

- Where in my life do I feel balance?

- Where in my life do I feel imbalance?

- How do I express myself in my career?

- How do I express myself in my health?

- How do I express myself in my relationships?

- If I know my purpose now, what actions can I take
  to further it?

Remember, you might not be able to fully 'hear' your purpose just yet, and that's OK. But you *will* get there; because you do 100 per cent have a purpose.

Mantras for Motivation

Incoming: Mantras are a bit like affirmations, but there's a difference. They are also a form of meditation and, in my experience, they are incredibly powerful. Mantras help to quieten the mind, create space between your thoughts and allow you to let go of any thoughts that are causing you stress, frustration and anger. Mantras can also help you to change destructive thoughts into constructive ones.

SELF-CARE ACTION:
Mantras to the rescue!

Each morning throughout this month, set your timer for three minutes before you need to get out of bed. Pick the mantra that seems most appropriate for the coming day. Then close your eyes and, as you silently repeat your chosen mantra to yourself, start to meditate on it: start to see the mantra happening, start to believe it, start to feel its presence within you. I guarantee that your mantra will then pop into your head several times throughout your day, even when you're not meditating.

It becomes so ingrained that you hear it over and over. And that's super-empowering!

Mantra 1

'I know my purpose, even though part of me might be frightened to know it.'

Often, we *do* know our purpose, but our self-esteem is so low that we condition ourselves to believe that we don't know it – that we don't know what we're doing with our lives. We do this to avoid the truth, to avoid the purpose that just might be tugging at us.

Mantra 2

'I'm now open to see why I'm unclear and I want to be shown the reasons.'

Start to tell your true, authentic self that you're ready. You accept that things right now seem a bit fuzzy and that's OK. But you're equally ready to be shown the reasons why. Perhaps it's because at some point in your past you were told that no one has a purpose, or that only the 'greats' of this world have one. And this kind of negative talk has affected you so much that you're sending yourself conflicting messages. Use this mantra to bring to the surface those types of stories. Let go of anything in the past that told you you don't have a purpose, for once and for all. Once you get rid of that stigma, things will start to open up. You will see within yourself much more clearly.

Mantra 3

'Fear is normal. I'm allowed to feel fear and any other emotion that comes with recognising my purpose.'

As we discussed in Month Ten, fear is normal, and you can use it to your advantage, to fuel, empower, dig deeper and find your purpose. You can still be scared. That's allowed. Heck, I'm still scared, but I use the fear and, in turn, I create courage to live my purpose.

Mantra 4

'My purpose may shift throughout my life, and that's OK.'

Many of us think we have just one purpose in life. And for some, that might be the case. But others might go through a lot of changes in their lives, and embark on many different paths headed towards different destinations. And yes, that is totally normal and OK.

The important thing is to remind yourself that whatever your journey is and wherever it takes you, you are on that path for a reason. You still have a purpose, no matter where you go. Changing paths can be difficult, but you can make this change a little bit easier if you give yourself permission to let go of what might have been and instead welcome what's coming next.

These mantras aren't magic, but they are useful and will help in the long run, by making space between your thoughts to help clarify and fulfil your purpose in life.

As I've been saying over and over throughout this chapter, every single one of us on this planet has a purpose, whether we realise it yet or not. It can be within your volunteering, your career, your parenting or any other part of your life.

SELF-CARE ACTION: The three lists

One of the best ways to discover your purpose is to make lists and connect the dots. And sometimes pieces come together that you never thought possible, so keep an open mind.

Love list

What are the things you love? I'm not just talking about making a list of things you love 'to do'. I'm talking about the things you love, including foods, places you love to travel to, your kids, your job, your partner, your parents, animals, history, culture, music and, of course, the things you love to do as well. Get specific. And once you've done this, take a step back and see how all of the things you love might connect together. Let your inspiration and your pen go crazy. Be creative!

Easy list

Now that you've made your Love List, you're going to make another list. The Easy List. Write down the things you do with ease – things that come naturally to you. (We touched upon this in an earlier chapter so it should be getting easy too!) What you do with ease in your everyday life is likely to be somehow connected to your purpose. For example, public speaking is something that comes very easily to me. I never get nervous speaking in front of a crowd, whether large or small. In fact, I love it! So I can look at this and connect it back to my purpose: I want to make sure people feel good about themselves; to do that, I must communicate that message to them, and even hug them. (I love a good hug!)

Don't overlook these talents – yes, the things that come easily to you *are* talents. So don't dismiss them and think everyone else can do them with ease too, because what comes easily to you isn't necessarily easy for everyone else. But by building on what does come easily to you, you have the opportunity to help others and to even touch many people's lives in ways you never thought possible.

What comes naturally to you? What do you do with ease?

Past list

Lastly, comes your Past List. The very struggles, heartbreaks and disappointments you've managed to move through in your life often become part of the tapestry that is your purpose. By looking at those 'life experiences' (as I like to call them) that you've success-fully conquered and learned from – and perhaps even changed as a result of – you can find a new perspective on life.

List your struggles, heartbreaks and disappointments that you've successfully conquered and learned from here:

Remember what I've been saying throughout this month, about passion and purpose going hand in hand. I like to think of them as the very best of friends. And by looking at your Love, Easy and Past Lists, you'll start to see all the dots connecting together.

There are countless experiences and adventures waiting to be discovered, and so many of them could inspire you to change your life for the better. Look for things that you are interested in and also open yourself up to trying things that you have no previous experience of or interest in. You never know what could come from doing so!

There is much to be gained, emotionally and spiritually, by embracing positive change and trying new things. You will meet new people, expand your knowledge and enjoy fresh challenges. Not every single new adventure will contribute in a huge way to living your life with more purpose, but there is something to be gained from every effort.

Month Twelve

Enhance Your Happiness
and Spread It Around

If with a pure mind a person speaks
or acts, happiness follows them like a
never-departing shadow.

BUDDHA

We all have muscles that we try very hard to make tougher and healthier and, yes, happier! We work our triceps, biceps, quads, hamstrings and hearts, stretching, building and feeding them to make them stronger, which, in turn, makes them – and us – happier. Well, it's the same with our happiness: we also need to work what I like to call our happiness muscle.

Work Your Happiness Muscle

We are solely in charge of creating, feeding and building our own happiness. And when we do this, we feel great. But it also feels great to spread this happiness to other people too.

People who are happy – and I mean the genuinely happy people – make a conscious decision to be happy, no matter what. Too often we choose to feed our unhappiness, by saying negative things, such as, 'Today was the worst day ever'. But this month we are going to choose to feed our happiness instead, by feeding and working our happiness muscles.

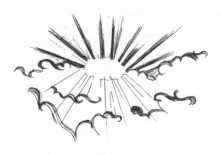

Happiness for Health

Research has shown that people who are happy are physically, emotionally and mentally healthier. And more successful! However, these genuinely happy people have to work at it. They weren't born feeling happy all of the time. Their happiness isn't something that they caught or picked up from their success, their gadgets, their fame, friends or money. It comes from within, and is something that is accessible to everyone.

We all have, at our core, a happiness muscle just waiting to be worked and strengthened.

The Happy People

You can always spot the happy ones: they have that infectious energy and that envious glow. They are a pleasure to be around and that's why others seem to be attracted to them. But how did they get this way? And how do they hold on to their happiness?

The truth is that becoming a genuinely happy person and maintaining this positive frame of mind is no small challenge. However, one thing's for sure, and that is that their happiness is the result of consistent dedication to self-care and focusing on internal, instead of external, influences. I know that can be difficult at times, but it's what we've been doing in this book for almost a year now: creating habits and making commitments to self-care, and now it's time for the end result, which is our own true happiness!

What's Holding You Back From Happiness?

What is it that genuinely happy people do? To find the answer to this burning question, I went on a personal mission, dissecting and analysing the mindsets and behaviour of seemingly genuinely happy people. And wow – was it an eye-opening experience! Here's what I found:

Comparisons

When a person is happy, there is much less need for them to compare their lives to those of other people. They simply acknowledge that they are happy with the choices that they have made in life, and they are completely satisfied with what they have and who they are, no matter what anyone else has or is.

Regrets

Living in the past is a no-no for happy people. They don't waste their time dwelling on regrets; the words 'dwelling' and 'regrets' don't exist in their vocabulary. Instead of wasting time thinking about past mistakes, happy people focus their energy on creating a positive and happy future for themselves.

Complaints

Complaining about something that has happened doesn't get anybody anywhere, and it is certainly not a habit that happy people adopt. Focusing on the positive, rather than the negative, is an essential mindset for a better and happier future.

Criticising others

Criticising other people is an activity that only unhappy people engage in and is generally a sign of deep insecurities. Happy people care about the well-being and happiness of others, and have no interest in emotionally damaging anyone else.

Trying to change others

Happy people don't try to change the behaviour or attitudes of other people. Doing this shows that the perpetrator is actually frustrated with themselves! When someone accepts themselves, they accept others, regardless of their perceived flaws.

Personal growth

Happy people consolidate their happiness by making time to work towards their dreams, goals and ambitions. They live their passions and give all their energy to the things and people that are important to them and make them happy.

Procrastinating

Wasting time is a behaviour seen frequently in unhappy people. They procrastinate and are reluctant to make any kind of positive changes in their own lives. Happy people stay present and appreciate every moment for the gift that it is, knowing that this is essential to a happy and emotionally satisfying life.

Seeking approval

Happy people do not need to seek the approval of others because this judgement is not important to them. They understand that all of the choices they have made in life are for their own good and disapproval or negative comments from others do not stop them from living their truth.

Overthinking

If a person spends too much time in their own head, allow-

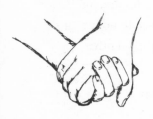

ing thoughts to spiral out of control, then depression, anxiety and sadness are bound to prevail. Happy people combat negative thoughts with positive ones.

Happiness Starts With Us

When I've asked my yoga students and some of my clients what truly makes them happy, the answers have, of course, varied. But they all had a similar theme: happiness starts with us. Happiness is not something you can buy or even buy into; it is not a gimmick or a trick.

Happiness is there. It's within our reach, but we need to understand how to create it.

I truly believe that happiness is much easier when we are healthy, and by that I don't just mean physically fit, but emotionally and mentally too. Over the past eleven months, you've learned some revolutionary habits, putting them into practice every single day, and while you may not have realised it, happiness is one of the many amazing side effects of the work you've been doing here. How much happier do you feel in this final month?

Creating your own happiness can range from journalling, to a new romance, to letting go of a toxic relationship, to doing a yoga practice, to stating affirmations, to meditation and everything else you've learned over the past twelve months. But for me, my big takeaway, after incorporating all of these small moments of self-care into my own life, is that all of the things you choose to adopt must become a habit – you have to do them consistently.

More Ideas for Creating Happiness

Creating happiness as a habit is a worthwhile journey. Added to what you've already done over these past eleven months, there are a few more small steps and habits to incorporate:

Trust your instincts

Your heart will always be a better guide than your head. This may conflict with advice that you've received before, but when was the last time you benefited from stressing out and overanalysing something? Trusting the way that your heart feels about a situation will keep you in touch with your feelings and enable you to live a life that is true to you.

Enjoy the journey

Constantly striving to reach some future destination where you believe happiness lies will often leave you disappointed with the present. When you accept that life is all about the journey, then you begin to enjoy each step that you take. It is always great to work towards and accomplish a goal, but try not to place too much emphasis on the importance of the future and learn to live in the now.

Embrace your curiosity

Fear of the unknown is a serious barrier to happiness, and encouraging yourself to take risks will help you to discover the things that will make you happy. If something arouses your curiosity, then make the time to check it out; you've nothing to lose and, possibly, a new passion to gain.

Forgive your flaws

Even happy people can sometimes fall victim to negative feelings, such as judgement, jealousy and anger. The difference is that they acknowledge that they have felt these things, and then make the conscious decision not to dwell on them. When you experience a negative thought – about yourself or others – it's totally fine to explore it before releasing it from your mind and forgiving yourself for it.

Invite change

Being happy with your life doesn't mean that it has to stay exactly the same. It's OK to change your mind about a situation or another person, and to let this change unfold naturally. Inviting change into your life should be seen as taking a step towards a new adventure or experience, and never as a step backwards.

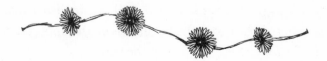

Let go
When something is dragging you and your mood down, the best thing you can do is simply to let go of it. If something or someone is making you unhappy then they are no longer serving you well, and walking away is a sign of strength and self-love, not weakness. You will notice that happy people have no time for this kind of negativity and instead surround themselves with positivity in many forms.

SELF-CARE ACTION:
How to spread happiness

Once you have begun to cultivate your own happiness, one of the best things you can do is to spread it around. Doing so not only helps others to find their happiness, but also encourages your positivity to continue thriving.

The following are simple ways to spread your happiness to other people:

- Be kind to everyone you meet during each day.
- Give often – whether this is gifts to friends, compliments to strangers, donations to charity, advice to those who ask for it . . .
- Reserve time and patience for those who really need your help.
- Share your struggles to inspire others and be honest about your experiences.

There are so many different creative ways to make other people happy, and you probably have lots of ideas of your own – list your favourite ones here:

Find the time to put these ideas into practice and notice the difference it makes to your own life, as well as the lives of others.

Anne's Story

One of my students created a great exercise to start to create her own happiness. Here's Anne's happiness story:

'Despite having lived in the UK and USA for the past fourteen years, as an Australian I struggle with the dark, grey, cold months of winter, particularly February. I crave light and sunshine and find British winters almost claustrophobic. I wanted to do something to keep myself and my thoughts positive, especially during this dark and grey period.

'I read an article about this thing called a "Jar of Awesome". It sounded like an excellent practice for both myself and my family – something that would lift February for me.

'The concept is quite simple: you designate a jar, and when something awesome or good happens to you or something has made you feel good, you write it down on a slip of paper, fold it and put it in your jar. It's a way of checking in daily with all that you are grateful for and maintaining positive thoughts. On some days you may have nothing to add to the jar, while on others you may have lots of notes. The beauty of the jar is that when things are tough, you open it and remind yourself of all the good moments of your life.

'I decided to rope my whole family into this project – my husband and two daughters (aged five and seven) – and I have to say it has been a resounding success. Essentially, you are focusing on the good, even if it was small, and rerouting your neural pathways onto a positive track. It becomes a habit, and I can say for certain that, more often than not, it has helped us to take a positive outlook rather than what might have been the default negative point of view.

'I particularly loved the way it made my daughters think. They wrote things like, "I am so glad I don't have a fever any more" and, "My tooth is wobbly!" It surprised me, as they really thought about what they wanted to put in and, more importantly, tried to capture small moments of good, happiness or joy, rather than simply writing, "I got a new toy". We all noticed that even during this dark, grey month we were happier because we were creating more positive thoughts throughout our day.'

SELF-CARE ACTION: Jar of happiness

Perhaps you can involve your family, roommates or whoever you live with in this happiness habit-creating exercise. If you're going to include others, it's quite a nice idea either for each person to use different-coloured paper or a different-coloured pen or pencil.

Each day, write either one or many things down that made you happy. There might be days when you just feel you can't do it, and that's OK and normal. But what you can then do instead is to reach into your jar and pull out one or more of your previous happy thoughts to keep that positive thinking going, regardless of what kind of day you've had.

Using Mindfulness For Happiness

Mindfulness is based upon certain mental techniques, the origins of which are in ancient Buddhist teachings.

However, there certainly don't have to be any religious connotations attached to it. Mindfulness can help you to better process your thoughts and feelings and also to retain more control over your emotions.

The following are mindfulness-based concepts and actions that you can embrace to help you become a happier person.

1. Break negative cycles

Mindfulness can help to put a stop to negative thoughts in the moment that you are experiencing them. When you begin along an unhelpful train of thought, your mind is going to perpetuate this unhappy state of mind, and this can quickly become detrimental to your life in several ways. But you can create a mindset that is more concerned with the positive by choosing to disengage from negative thoughts and replacing them with positive ones or by physically doing something else in that moment to distract yourself.

2. Connect with others

As people, we are naturally inclined to be sociable beings and will often crave this kind of interaction when it is lacking. Mindfulness is a beautiful way to deepen our relationships with others, as well as to better enable us to form new bonds with like-minded people.

3. Create contentment

The technology that is all around us these days makes it easy to fall into the trap of thinking that we need to be constantly stimulated in order to be happy. In addition, many of us have also become prone to seeking the approval of others. However, we often have no control over this and it can leave us feeling that we are lacking something.

Mindfulness teaches you to embrace a new type of happiness that is not dependent in any way on external factors or circumstances. This happiness will take root from an inner sense of well-being – being happy with where you are right now – and from placing an emphasis on strong values and morals.

4. Express gratitude

We discussed gratitude in Month Five, but here is a reminder! Practising gratitude in a mindful way will help you to stay present. Taking the time to express gratitude and take stock of all the good things that you have in your life is a great way to reconnect to the present moment – and this is the essence of mindfulness. When you acknowledge all the reasons why you should be happy, you will naturally become more thankful for these things.

Expressing gratitude can be done in small spontaneous ways, such as stopping to really appreciate something in the present moment; or it can also be done in larger ways, such as sharing feelings of gratitude with someone who is a positive presence in your life.

Let's Get Away From Autopilot

We are all guilty, at least on occasion, of living our lives on autopilot, and when we do so, we miss out on those all-important moments of self-care.

Regardless of how busy you are, finding the time to practise mindfulness will mean you are choosing to consciously prioritise your overall well-being. Even the most routine of activities can be an opportunity to engage in a moment of mindfulness – and the potential is always there.

Happy daily tasks

All too often, unwarranted emphasis is placed on battling through our to-do lists. And when we view our daily tasks in this way, the list can seem never-ending. In fact, it can often feel as though every time you go to cross one thing off, two new tasks appear on the list! So how can we prevent this constant state of busyness and limit the extent to which these stresses impact on our lives, making us simply unhappy?

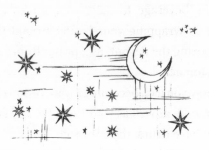

Let's take a look at some routine things that you, more than likely, do daily. I want to show how you can change your attitude towards them, and create a greater sense of well-being and happiness for yourself while doing them.

SELF-CARE ACTION:
Bringing mindfulness to your routine

Your morning coffee

If you begin your day with a coffee hit, or even if you prefer to have a tea or a green juice, then turning this simple act into a ritual is a great way to invite some mindfulness in.

- Pay full attention to your drink; shutting out any distractions is key here.
- Be still and be silent with your beverage of choice, and feel all of the sensations throughout your body as you drink it slowly.

- Allow the beverage to meet your senses through smelling it, wrapping your hands around the cup and savouring the flavour, as it passes from your lips to your stomach.
- Notice how you feel, becoming aware of any changes in your mood, as well as your thoughts and feelings, until you have drunk the last drop.

Taking a shower

Taking a shower can be a very sensual experience, but this is often missed in our haste to get ready in the morning.

- When you take your shower, make the time to feel the water on your body, and how it cleanses you emotionally as well as physically.
- Breathe in the scent of your soaps and creams as you use them, and feel how your body awakens as you wash from top to bottom.
- Visualisation is a great tool here, and imagining your stresses, anxieties and tensions being washed away as you shower can help you to start the day in a positive and happy frame of mind.

Mealtimes

Understanding each meal as a chance to really nourish yourself, and taking the time to truly enjoy it, will enhance every mealtime and turn it into a simple act of self-care.

- Eat a meal slowly.
- Appreciate the tastes, textures and flavours that it provides, allowing the beauty of mindfulness to unfold at each meal.
- Start to express gratitude for the nourishment that you are receiving.

Getting fit

Ask anyone who exercises and they will most likely tell you that they do it in order to get physically fit, by improving their stamina or enhancing their strength. However, adopting an approach to exercise that goes beyond building muscle, paying attention to your mental health and well-being, will allow you to gain a deeper satisfaction from each workout. In addition, you will become much more aware of the bigger picture, and understand the benefits of exercising far beyond the physical gains. Why not use positive affirmations as you work out to help truly create that happy mindset (see pages 47–54).

List your get-fit daily exercises and positive affirmations here:

Happiness is right here, in all of us and all around us. It's up to us now to create it – because the key to happiness lies within.

Moments of Self-care: 21-Day Challenge

Your twelve-month self-care journey may be at an end but I know you will have created some amazing habits, which you will carry through on a daily basis for the rest of your life. And remember, you can pick this book up anytime you need to revisit a particular month in order to re-establish that healthy habit. But I want to leave you with a self-care bonus: it's my self-care 21-day challenge that you can start immediately after completing these twelve months, or whenever you like.

Day One: An Exercise to Breathe Better Now

We are going to start Day One with our breath. This breathing exercise is simple and super-effective. It will help you to slow down, de-stress and prepare yourself for the day ahead.

- Count your breath for ten breaths. One round is an inhale and an exhale. Like this: inhale one, exhale one, inhale two, exhale two, inhale three, exhale three and so on.

- Now do another ten rounds, but you're going to count both the inhales and the exhales this time. So: inhale one, exhale two, inhale three, exhale four, all the way up to twenty.

- Once you complete the twenty counts, you are going to count again, but just your inhales for twenty, and this time counting down. So: inhale twenty, exhale, inhale nineteen, exhale, inhale eighteen, exhale and so on.

- Next, you are going to count your exhales up to twenty, like this: inhale, exhale one, inhale, exhale two, inhale, exhale three and so on all the way to twenty.

- And lastly, you are going to do another ten full rounds of breath, but counting down from ten. So, inhale ten, exhale ten, inhale nine, exhale nine, inhale eight, exhale eight and so on all the way down to one.

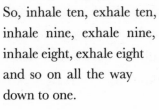

Day Two:
Positive Affirmations

We know from Month Four that saying a positive affirmation on a daily basis is great for our happiness and our
lives. So the positive affirmation for today is:

'I have everything I need right now to be happy.'

As you say this, start to visualise the things that you have
right now in your life to make you happy, then feel that
happiness starting to take shape in your body. And if you
say it multiple times today, that's even better!

Day Three: Happiness Tea Tonic

Get ready to feel happy with my happiness tea tonic. This
is my go-to tonic when I want to feel happy all day long.
And the good news is that all the ingredients used here are
ones you can keep on hand.

Makes 2 cups

1 ginger tea bag (or piece of peeled root ginger)
2 cups boiling water
½ cinnamon stick or a pinch of cinnamon
dash of cayenne pepper (optional)
1 tsp apple cider vinegar
1 orange slice

1–2 tsp honey (depending on how sweet you like it)

Use either a small teapot or an extra-large mug. Place the ginger tea bag or fresh ginger inside. Pour the boiling water into the mug/teapot and let it steep for 5 minutes. Give the tea bag a good squeeze and then remove it.

Add the cinnamon and cayenne (if using) and stir until combined. Next, add the vinegar, orange slice and honey. Stir again and enjoy.

This tea is great for encouraging feelings of happiness. Ginger contains a potent antioxidant known as gingerol, which will help to alleviate the effects of stress hormones in the body. Ginger in a hot tea is also a simple way to relieve stress, thanks to the calming scent. Plus, studies have shown that the scent of cinnamon can help to enhance feelings of calm and happiness, while its antibacterial properties can be effective in tackling the harmful bacteria in the gut that can contribute to depression.

Day Four: Mindset Shift

As we learned in Month Four, it is possible to change the limiting beliefs that you have about yourself. In doing so, you can rebuild your self-esteem and allow your confidence to thrive.

Grab your journal and pen and take ten minutes to write down one or two limiting beliefs about yourself that keep popping up in your head. For example, 'I'm not pretty enough', 'I'm not thin enough', 'I'm not clever enough'. You know what yours are. Next, you are going to rewrite them, reframing them in a positive way, so that you start to shift your mindset. So rather than saying, 'I'm not pretty enough', you write a sentence including two or three or more things about your appearance that are positive: 'My eyes are striking, I have wonderful hair and I like my feet'. If your limiting belief is, 'I'm not good enough', then your mindset-shift sentence should list two to three of your accomplish-ments (and yes, I know you have achieved a lot in your life). As you carry on with the rest of your day, allow these positive thoughts to override the negative ones.

Day Five:
Happiness Yoga Pose

This is my go-to I-want-to-feel-good-and-happy yoga pose that *anyone* can do *anytime*. I call it my Happiness Pose and I promise you that after you do this simple but super-effective pose, you will feel better and happier.

- Start out by lying down on the floor, close enough to a wall that you can put your legs up against it. Try to nuzzle your tailbone as close to the wall as possible (optional: put a book under your sacrum to get your hips higher than your heart).

- Put one hand on your heart and the other on your belly. Inhale for four counts, pressing your hand into your belly in order to expand your body with your breath. As you exhale, draw your belly towards the floor and try to exhale for five to six counts. Keep your eyes closed to calm the central nervous system.
- Stay in this position and repeat the breathing exercise for at least two minutes, silently repeating to yourself, 'I choose to create my own happiness'. If you need to, you can put a timer on for two minutes, but your mantra needs to be silently repeated, over and over again, until the two minutes are up.

When you do this Happiness Pose regularly, you should notice that your body feels healthier throughout each day too, which, of course, will make you happier.

Day Six: Candlelit Bath with Epsom Salts

How about splurging and buying yourself a gorgeous-smelling and calming candle today? Because no matter what your day was like, you're going to end it with a wonderful candlelit bath and some oh-so-good-for-you Epsom salts. Epsom salts work immediately as they are absorbed through the skin. As the magnesium ions enter your body they begin to relieve stress and enhance serotonin levels.

Magnesium can also provide a boost of energy without any negative side effects.

Make sure all electronic devices are switched off, dim the lights, light the candle, slip into your bath and allow the salts to be absorbed into your body. Close your eyes and stay there for fifteen to twenty minutes. During this time, visualise the type of day you want to have tomorrow ... and smile.

Day Seven: Replace TV Time with Reading Time

If you usually end your evenings watching TV – whether that's on your actual TV or on a computer screen – tonight you're going to switch it all off. Instead, you're going to read a book that inspires you, that motivates you, that makes you feel happy when you go to sleep. Try to read for thirty minutes before you turn off the light. Set a timer if you need to, but get those thirty minutes in, and even longer if you can. (So if you normally watch TV for an hour before bed, try to read for sixty minutes.) When you read something inspirational just before bed, you will fall asleep feeling happy inside, and are more likely to wake up still happy!

Day Eight: Healthy Supper Recipe with Shopping List

Cooking a meal for yourself, for your family or for your roommates is unbelievably rewarding. Cooking helps you to stay in the present moment because you have to pay attention to the recipe, the ingredients, the baking, the boiling, the frying and so on.

Here is one of my favourite plant-based recipes that is so good for you and so easy to make that you can't help but be happy while you prepare it, eat it and after you've finished it as your digestion system kicks in.

Coconut Vegetable Curry with Chickpeas

Serves 4

1 tbsp finely chopped fresh ginger

1½ tsp cumin seeds

1 tsp black mustard seeds

1 large sweet potato, cut into cubes

3 medium carrots, chopped

½ tsp turmeric

2 tsp coriander

1 tsp curry powder

1 tbsp tomato paste

400ml tin coconut milk

½ cup water

2 small courgettes, chopped

1 cup frozen peas or green beans
1 × 400g tin chickpeas, drained and rinsed
Handful fresh coriander leaves, chopped

In a large saucepan, heat 120ml water over a medium heat and add the ginger, cumin seeds and black mustard seeds; cook for 2 minutes or until the seeds begin to pop.

Add the sweet potato, carrots, turmeric, coriander and curry powder. Stir well and continue to cook for another minute or so.

Add the tomato paste, coconut milk and water and stir well. Simmer with the lid on for 5–10 minutes, until the sweet potato and carrots are almost cooked.

Add the courgettes and peas or beans and chickpeas. Cover again and simmer until all the vegetables are tender – about 6–7 minutes. Remove from the heat and stir in the chopped coriander. Serve with brown rice or quinoa.

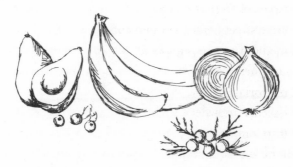

Day Nine: Walking Mindfully

Wherever you walk today – whether it's for a power walk or to get to the Tube or bus, pick up the kids from school, get to work or run your errands – you're going to do it mindfully.

Start to notice your feet, the shoes that you're wearing and the steps they are making heel to toe, over and over again. Forget about the destination during your walk. Forget about what you're going to do once you get there. If thoughts come into your mind, such as to-do lists or anything that takes you away from your walk, just bring your awareness back to your feet, back to your breath and back to the sights, smells and sounds surrounding you.

Day Ten: Move More With Little Effort

What do I mean by this? Well, if you're in your car today and have to run an errand, park the car in the farthest parking spot and walk from there to the shop. If you have a choice between taking a lift or walking up the stairs, take the stairs. Or, if an escalator is the only option, walk up it. If you have a meeting, make it a walking meeting. Even if you're taking public transport, perhaps you can walk to the next stop rather than the one that's closest to you. These are all little measures you can put in place to allow you to move more without too much effort. We often forget about these things, but they are so simple to incorporate.

Day Eleven: Power Posture

Going into a tough meeting? Need to have a difficult conversation with someone? Worried about feeling alone and out of place at an event? Or surrounded by energy vampires? Well, today you're going to strike a pose. You're going to stand tall, proud and confident because your posture can change the way you feel about yourself.

Simply take your shoulders up, back and down and breathe right into the space you've just created across your collarbones and into your heart.

Day Twelve: Healthy Breakfast Recipe

Let's start the day on a happy, healthy note with a super-yummy, nutritious and energising breakfast.

Blueberry Almond Oatmeal

Serves 1–2

1 cup thick rolled oats
240ml water
pinch of sea salt
maple syrup or agave nectar, to taste
blueberries, fresh or frozen, to taste
ground almonds, a small handful
cinnamon, a dash or more

Place the oats, water, and sea salt in a medium saucepan. Turn the heat to medium and cook until the mixture begins to bubble, then turn the heat to low.

Continue stirring until the oatmeal is thick and cooked, about 10 minutes.

Divide between serving bowls, top with a little maple syrup or agave nectar, a handful of blueberries and a table-spoon or two of ground almonds. Sprinkle with cinnamon.

Note: if you want to make this the night before and keep it in your fridge, you can. You don't even have to cook the oats. Just soak them in the water the night before and they will be lovely and soft in the morning.

Day Thirteen: Positive Music

Oh, the power of music! We all know that music can lift our mood, creating happiness in our everyday lives. Well, today you are going to compile your own happiness playlist. Get on your iTunes, your Spotify or head to any musical website. Download around twelve songs – which will be approximately one hour's worth of music. All of the songs should be ones that make you smile when you hear them.

Play your happy music *all* day today. Listen to it in your earphones or blast it anytime. Be sure to listen to all twelve of your happy songs throughout your day!

Day Fourteen: Five-minute Relaxation Technique

This relaxation technique is something I often do at the end of my yoga classes or workshops. But you don't need my voice to do it. You can do it on your own – it's very simple and effective and makes you feel great afterwards.

- Lie down somewhere comfortable, warm and quiet.
- In your mind, start to trace around your body and observe how each body part feels, without judgement. Begin with the right hand and trace around your body until you connect back to the right hand, finishing at the place where you started. You might need to stay on one body part longer than the others if that part of the body needs a bit more breath, a bit more attention, because it is hurting physically or emotionally.

Do this as many times as you need to today to really allow yourself to calm down, find peace and relax.

Day Fifteen: Practising Gratitude

As we have now learned, appreciating what we have is one of the keys to a healthier, happier life.

Showing gratitude can boost your satisfaction with your life, improve your mental health and well-being, help you sleep better and stick with your workout routine, make you more optimistic, increase self-esteem and energy levels, relax better and simply makes you feel good.

Write down three things in your journal that you're grateful for. Do this first thing in the morning and before you go to bed at night.

Day Sixteen: Healthy Snack Recipe

You can take this to work with you, on the road or just have it on hand at home today. It's delicious.

Pea Guacamole

1 cup frozen peas, thawed
1 avocado, peeled and pitted
2 large cloves garlic, crushed
juice of 1 lime
1 tsp ground cumin
1 tomato, chopped
2 spring onions, chopped
large handful chopped fresh coriander
1–2 tsp red chilli flakes (optional)
sea salt and freshly ground pepper, to taste

Put the peas, avocado, garlic, lime juice and cumin in a food processor and process until smooth.

Scrape the mixture into a bowl and stir in the tomato,

spring onions, coriander and red chilli flakes (if using). Season to taste.

Cover and refrigerate for at least 30 minutes to allow the flavours to blend. Serve with wholegrain rice cakes or raw veggies.

Day Seventeen: Flow Your Breath – Alternate-nostril Breathing

As you discovered in Month Seven, alternate-nostril breathing is a great way to balance your nervous system. Most of us have an overly active sympathetic nervous system – you know, that fight/flight/freeze stress response (see page 37). And we'd like to get more into the parasympathetic nervous system, the rest-and-digest relaxation response (see page 50). Breathing through your right nostril is connected to your sympathetic nervous system, and breathing through your left nostril is connected to your parasympathetic nervous system. So today I'd like you to get more balanced by doing the Alternate-nostril Breathing exercise on page 148.

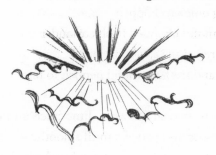

Day Eighteen: Feel-good Yoga Pose to Do Anywhere

Did you know that a simple forward fold is a) a yoga pose and b) one of the best poses you can do to make yourself feel so, so good? Plus, you can do it anytime, anywhere, in just your regular clothes – yes, even 'work' clothes.

- Start with your feet at least as wide apart as your hips, even wider, if it feels more comfortable.
- As you inhale, lift the chest up towards the sky to help lengthen the spine.
- As you exhale, hinge at the hips and bend your upper body over your lower body. Let your arms go. If you need to bend the knees to help soften the hamstrings, then take a gentle bend in your knees. When you go into your forward fold, try to stay in it for at least two minutes, while breathing in for four counts and out for six.

There are some great health benefits to this pose. In the two minutes you're folding forward, and with this breath count, you'll get in about twelve really good breaths while the blood is flowing to your face and head for mental clarity and emotional stability.

Day Nineteen: Green Smoothie Recipe

Today, enjoy this simple, so good smoothie – this recipe will definitely put a smile on your face.

Happiness smoothie

1 good handful fresh spinach
1 good handful fresh kale
small handful walnuts
1 small cucumber, peeled
1 pear, peeled and cored
1 small banana
240ml almond milk or plant-based milk of your choice

Combine the spinach, kale, walnuts, cucumber, pear and banana with half the almond milk in a blender.

With the blender running, add the remaining almond milk. Whizz until smooth, serve and slurp!

Day Twenty: Meditate

Improving your energy, focusing your mind and reducing your stress levels are some of the many benefits of meditation, as you now know. Use this five-minute meditation whenever you want more energy, need to really focus on tasks or deadlines or if you're just feeling incredibly stressed out.

- Find a comfortable spot to sit (and oh, by the way, you can even do this in the office). Don't control your breath, just continue to let your body breathe for you.
- As you inhale, silently repeat to yourself, 'My whole body', and as you exhale, say, 'is relaxed'.
- Inhale: 'Let'; exhale: 'go'.
- Inhale: 'I take'; exhale: 'care of me'.
- Inhale: 'My whole body'; exhale: 'is focused'.
- Inhale: 'My whole body'; exhale: 'is at peace'.
- Inhale: 'My whole body'; exhale: 'is calm'.
- Inhale: 'My whole body'; exhale: 'is healthy'.
- Inhale: 'My whole body'; exhale: 'is happy'.

Day Twenty-one: New, Positive Happiness Habits

Hooray! This is the last day of your 21-Day Self-care Challenge! And to go out on a high, you are going to choose eight habits from the above and incorporate them into your day today. For example, you might start the day with a Happiness Tea Tonic and Happiness Yoga Pose, followed by Walking Mindfully, your Breathe Better Now exercise and Healthy Supper Recipe, then Replace TV Time with Reading Time, a Candlelit Bath with Epsom Salts and Practising Gratitude. And that's it!

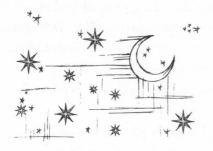

Final Thoughts

I am confident that with the tools, resources, tips and guidance that I have shared in this book you are now equipped to lead a life filled with good health, happiness, passion, purpose, courage and boundless positivity! Your energy will be elevated, your enthusiasm boundless and you will have much more focus for whatever you set out to achieve. And not only will all of these changes be apparent to you, I am certain that others in your life will start to notice them, too.

So, one last thing before I go: on my wrist, I wear a bracelet with my own mantra engraved on it. It reads: 'She needed a hero so that's what she became'. My hope for you is that through this year of self-care and focusing on you, you too will have become your very own *superhero*.

Appendix: Seven-day Food Diary

Keeping track of what you eat is a great way to make sure you are including enough of the anxiety-busting foods that I have mentioned earlier.

The seven-day food diary overleaf is designed for you to record everything that you eat during the next week (Alternatively, put together something similar in your diary or journal). Once you have reached the end of the week, you can look back and determine if you are getting enough of the good stuff in. It can also be helpful to see if you are consuming too much of the things that may exacerbate feelings of anxiety, such as caffeine and sugar.

As well as writing down what you eat each day, make a note of your feelings after each meal. This can help you become aware of how certain foods help or hinder your mood.

Monday	Tuesday	Wednesday	Thursday
Breakfast			
Lunch			
Dinner			
Snacks			
Drinks			

Friday	Saturday	Sunday

References

Introduction

https://www.mindbodygreen.com/0-13665/
   why-self-care-isnt-selfish.html

Month Two

http://www.medicalnewstoday.com/articles/299142.php

http://www.webmd.com/balance/stress-management/
   effects-of-stress-on-your-body

https://www.sciencedaily.com/releases/2012/11/121119163258.htm

http://www.dailymail.co.uk/femail/article-2938722/
   How-yoga-calms-mind-ll-help-beat-stress-anxiety-
   depression-without-popping-pills.html

Month Three

http://www.digitalresponsibility.org/health-and-technology/

https://www.globalhealingcenter.com/natural-health/
   10-shocking-facts-health-dangers-wifi/

https://www.rfsafe.com/cell-phone-radiation-exposure-
    increases-using-wired-hands-free-headsets/

https://www.theatlantic.com/health/archive/2014/11/
    what-texting-does-to-the-spine/382890/

https://techcrunch.com/2014/04/01/mobile-app-usage-
    increases-in-2014-as-mobile-web-surfing-declines/

http://www.apa.org/monitor/2017/03/cover-disconnected.aspx

https://www.health.harvard.edu/staying-healthy/
    blue-light-has-a-dark-side

Month Four

https://www.psychologytoday.com/articles/200306/
    our-brains-negative-bias

Month Five

https://www.theguardian.com/society/2016/jun/06/women-
    twice-as-likely-as-men-to-experience-anxiety-research-finds

https://www.fool.com/retirement/2016/11/14/are-your-
    personal-finance-woes-impacting-your-job.aspx

http://americanaddictioncenters.org/alcoholism-treatment/anxiety/

http://articles.mercola.com/sites/articles/archive/2015/01/19/
    magnesium-deficiency.aspx

https://www.psychologytoday.com/blog/
    evolutionary-psychiatry/201303/yoga-ba-gaba

Month Ten

http://www.theodore-roosevelt.com/trsorbonnespeech.html

Notes